An Introduction to

DIAGNOSTIC NEUROLOGY

A COURSE OF INSTRUCTION FOR STUDENTS

An Introduction to

DIAGNOSTIC NEUROLOGY

A COURSE OF INSTRUCTION FOR STUDENTS

BY

STEWART RENFREW

Neurologist, Royal Infirmary, Glasgow

ILLUSTRATIONS
BY
ROBIN CALLANDER

VOLUME II

SECOND EDITION
REPRINT

CHURCHILL LIVINGSTONE
EDINBURGH AND LONDON
1974

CHURCHILL LIVINGSTONE
Medical Division of Longman Group Limited

Represented in the United States of America by
Longman Inc., New York, and by associated
companies, branches and representatives throughout the world.

First edition 1962
Second edition 1967
Reprinted 1974

ISBN 0 443 00410 2

Printed in Hong Kong by
Yu Luen Offset Printing Factory Ltd.

INTRODUCTION TO PART III

INTRACRANIAL diseases are so numerous and cerebral disorders so varied and subtle that it is unreasonable to expect the student to attain anything more than a superficial knowledge. Rather than offer the student a multitude of facts it is better to give him some generalisations which will allow him to infer intracranial lesions confidently, although the identification of the precise type and exact site may elude him. In following this plan much detail has, therefore, been omitted and disorders of cranial nerves, for example, which seem to be an obsession with examiners, have been played down.

Again, as an aid to learning, diseases have been divided into two groups. The first group, which includes neoplasms and cerebro-vascular accidents, is easily taught and learned for there is no shortage of patients. The second group includes some rather rare conditions and it is unlikely that demonstrations of the entire group can be arranged for each class of students. Visits to Psychiatric units, however, should compensate for the lack of suitable patients in the general medical wards.

Chapters on Psychosomatic Disorders and the Electro-encephalogram have been included for the sake of completeness. Psychosomatic Disorders are usually taught by psychiatrists and, since their views are rarely enthusiastically accepted by general physicians, it seemed advisable to be critical of the psychiatrist's approach and to offer an alternative in its place. The chapter on the Electro-encephalogram is used as an excuse to emphasise, if emphasis at this stage is needed, the distinction between evidence and inference. The Electro-encephalogram will probably remain a mystery to students, no matter how it is taught, and the most that can be hoped for is that they will learn to use the test with some discretion.

Part of the teaching time of the third term should be spent in the neurological out-patient clinic for it is only here that the student will gain experience in seizures, head-aches and a wide variety of functional disorders of the nervous system.

CONTENTS

PART III—THIRD TERM

CEREBRAL SIGNS
AND INTRACRANIAL DISEASES

CEREBRAL SIGNS
AND INTRACRANIAL DISEASES

CHAPTER XIX

THE LANGUAGE OF EMPIRICAL SCIENCE

Cause and effect

The terms ' cause ' and ' effect' are used a great deal by everyone but few people would be prepared to define them. Let us see what we can make of this difficult problem of definition. In the general proposition

$$\text{Objects called } A \text{ which have } x \xrightarrow[m]{n} \text{have } y$$

we see that the properties are divided into two bundles and we have therefore no alternative but to call one the cause of the other. Thus we would say that x is the cause of y or that y is the cause of x. It may then be asked if the terms ' cause ' and ' effect' can be applied to the x and y of every correlative proposition. Certainly not, as the following example shows.

$$\text{People with blue eyes } \xrightarrow[100]{99} \text{sleep well.}$$

Despite the high probability of the correlation we could not suppose that blue eyes cause sleep or that sleep causes blue eyes. It would therefore appear that sometimes we can call x the cause of y, or *vice versa*, and sometimes not. What then are the rules? The rules governing the use of words are not, of course, natural laws but are simply those imposed by common usage. Our problem then is to discover how people in general use the words ' cause ' and 'effect'. An inquiry into the use of the words leads, it seems, to the following definition.

> A property is called a cause when its addition (to x) increases* the probability, or its removal (from x) decreases the probability of the property (y), called the effect.

Some examples given in diagrammatic form will make this clear.

who are living in Glasgow $\xrightarrow[10,000]{1}$ are dead a month later.

People

and have pneumonia $\xrightarrow[10]{1}$ are dead a month later.

Conclusion: Pneumonia is a cause of death.

who have pneumonia $\xrightarrow[10]{7}$ are alive a month later.

People

and get penicillin $\xrightarrow[10]{9}$ are alive a month later.

Conclusion: Penicillin is a cause of survival.

who have a large pleural effusion $\xrightarrow[10]{8}$ are breathless.

People

and have the fluid removed $\xrightarrow[10]{2}$ are breathless.

Conclusion: A large pleural effusion is a cause of breathlessness.

---

* The fact that a cause changes probability implies that the cause precedes the effect.

The definition of cause can now be given in general terms.

$$\text{Objects called } A \begin{cases} \text{which have } z \xrightarrow{\frac{n}{m}} \text{have } y. \\ \text{which have } z+x \xrightarrow{\frac{n+q}{m}} \text{have } y. \end{cases}$$

Conclusion: x is the cause of y.

$$\text{Objects called } A \begin{cases} \text{which have } z+x \xrightarrow{\frac{n}{m}} \text{have } y. \\ \text{which have } z \xrightarrow{\frac{n-q}{m}} \text{have } y. \end{cases}$$

Conclusion: x is the cause of y.

You will see from these diagrams that two propositions are required if a property is to be called a cause. It is also worth noting that when we call a property a cause we habitually, for the sake of brevity, no doubt, make no reference to the properties z to which the causal property has been added. For example, when we say that rubbing a match on a rough surface causes it to ignite we are leaving our listeners to assume that the match is dry. Clearly a certain property x will only act as a cause in certain circumstances z. Perhaps you may remember from your schooldays a mathematical definition to the effect that x is the logarithm of y to the base a. This may be written as follows.

$$x = \log_a y$$

The cause of an effect can be written in the same way.

$$x = \text{cause}_z y$$

Of course there is nothing mathematical about cause and effect but the little equation is a useful reminder that a causal property cannot be considered in isolation from other properties.

The introduction of causal properties now gives us two kinds of correlative propositions which may be called causal and non-causal. The following propositions are examples.

non-causal

People with blue eyes $\xrightarrow{\frac{99}{100}}$ sleep well.

non-causal

People with headache $\xrightarrow{\frac{1}{10,000}}$ have a brain tumour.

causal

People with a brain tumour $\xrightarrow{\frac{8}{10}}$ have headache.

In pursuing scientific research we have to aim at both kinds of propositions. Obviously we have to make sufficient observations to allow us to infer brain tumour from headache and, at the same time, we have to establish brain tumour as a cause of headache if we are to produce a cure —a cure that is, in the sense of removing the cause.

At first sight it may seem, assuming the above definition to be correct, that it is an easy matter to prove that certain properties are causal. Unfortunately it is very difficult. In practice it is almost impossible to add a property without adding many others or to remove a property without removing many others. For example, in giving an injection of penicillin you add much more to the patient than the penicillin itself. You add yourself to start with and the various aspects of your behaviour towards the patient. Next there is the needle, the solvent which contains the penicillin, the pain, the fear perhaps, and so on. In removing a tooth you remove some body tissue apart from the tooth itself and also you may remove anxiety. If this sounds rather absurd you should ask a clinician who has assessed a new drug to tell you about the difficulties he encountered. He will no doubt tell you that, in his research, the fortuitous addition of properties made it difficult for him to decide whether the property he intentionally added (that is, the drug) was actually the one that raised the probability of the inference. He will add that, in order to solve this problem, he had to enumerate all the properties which were added unavoidably in excess of the causal property (the drug) which was under investigation and that he then had to add these to patients who were not receiving the drug. Thus, in a drug trial, two groups of patients are investigated, one group receiving the drug and the other a dummy pill which is identical to the drug pill except that the drug itself is lacking. Moreover, to make the conditions as identical as possible in the two groups, the person giving the treatment must not be allowed to know which are the genuine pills in case his attitude to the individuals of the two groups should be different. In clinical language the patients who receive the dummy pills are called the control group.

The temporal sequence of cause and effect should not be given too much emphasis. Nevertheless, a cause usually seems more convincing when the property, thought to be the effect, follows immediately, for there is no time for other properties to be added or removed accidentally. When there is a long delay there is ample opportunity for other properties to be added or removed with the result that at the end of an experiment it may not be clear what part the property, which is under investigation, has played in changing the probability of the inference.

While the rapid succession of cause and effect is rather satisfying, there is the danger that the mere temporal juxtaposition of two properties, especially if often repeated, leads you to name the first as the cause of the second. For example, five minutes after I rise in the morning my neighbour's alarm clock rings. Is my rising the cause of the ringing? This problem is easily answered if you remember that two correlative propositions are required before a particular property can be called a cause. Even then, dramatic events may sway your judgment. There was once a scientist who was so impressed with the time relationship of volcanoes and epidemics that he concluded that the first was the cause of the second.

Apart from these remarks you must realise that, in identifying cause, close attention must be given to the time relations of properties. Consider the following propositions.

$$\text{with headache} \xrightarrow{\frac{1}{10,000}} \text{have a brain tumour.}$$

People

$$\text{and a hemiplegia} \xrightarrow{\frac{1}{100}} \text{have a brain tumour.}$$

It appears from this diagram that hemiplegia causes brain tumour, a conclusion which is absurd. What has gone wrong? The truth is that if hemiplegia was added to a group of people, none of whom had brain tumour, brain tumours would not develop. To avoid confusion the following rather obvious rule must be observed.

> To establish a property as a cause the proportion having the inference must be known before the property is added or removed.

If the rule had been observed in the above example, it would have been found that, of the patients who had headache and a hemiplegia, 1 in 100 had a brain tumour before the hemi-plegia was added.

This takes us to a difficulty which bedevils clinical work. In the investigation of the cause of pathological processes we are not at liberty, for ethical reasons, to add and remove properties indiscriminately. We can show that pathological abnormalities are the causes of symptoms and signs by removing them but this, of course, has nothing to do with finding the cause of the pathological abnormalities themselves. In research work, therefore, we often have to be content to be spectators in what are called experiments designed by nature. This is a profitable pursuit although difficult and often disappointing since it is seldom clear in what order properties appear.

Irritating as these difficulties are we should not be tempted into speculation about causal relations unless such speculation leads to experiment and observation. Unfor-tunately many clinicians are content to speculate freely and a feeling of conviction about their speculations is con-sidered to be a sort of verification of causal relations. I have changed Descartes' famous phrase ' I think, therefore I am ' to read ' *I think, therefore I am right* ' to describe this attitude of mind. To be sure that a property is a cause is not proof that it is a cause.

So far a difficulty has been ignored and it is this. How much change must occur in a probability before a property, which has been added or removed, can be called a cause? Here is an example.

$$\text{People}\begin{cases} \text{who have pneumonia} \xrightarrow{\frac{80}{100}} \text{survive.} \\ \\ \text{and take aspirin} \xrightarrow{\frac{82}{100}} \text{survive.} \end{cases}$$

Does the slight change in the probability justify calling aspirin a cause of survival, or, in other words, that it is a justifiable form of treatment of pneumonia? It has probably occurred to you that, in every series of 100 patients with pneumonia who do not have aspirin, it is unlikely that exactly 80 will survive. Perhaps in one series 75 patients will survive and in another 85 patients. The problem, it seems, is to decide when a probability produced by the addition or removal of a property is outwith the range of expected probabilities in a number of series in which the property is neither added nor removed. When the probability is well outside the normal range there is no difficulty, but otherwise the problem is acute and statistical methods have to be employed.

Some people claim that a cause should increase the probability of an effect to certainty when it is added, and reduce it to zero when it is removed. Such causes are sometimes called sufficient and necessary causes respectively. There is therefore room for considerable variation in the way people use the words ' cause ' and ' effect ' for, at one extreme, there are those who demand only a small but statistically significant change in probabilities while, at the other extreme, there are those who demand a large change. However, although there is no agreement about cause and effect, and probably never will be, you should have clear ideas yourself of how you are going to use these words. Do not change your definitions from moment to moment, for not only will you confuse other people but you will thoroughly confuse yourself.

As an exercise make up pairs of propositions (if you can!) which would justify the following common statements.

The tubercle bacillus causes human pulmonary tuberculosis.

Morphia kills pain.

Peptic ulcers are due to worry.

Heavy smoking causes bronchial carcinoma.

Exercise protects the heart from infarctions.

Multiple causes

Although we may say that x is the cause of y to the base z, it would also be correct to say that all the components of z are acting as causes. Thus in the example of the match, dryness and oxygen have as much right to be called causes as the rubbing although, of course, as components of z, they are taken for granted. It would seem, therefore, that one effect has several simultaneous causes and these may be called co-existent causes. Causes, however, may be multiple in another sense, for a cause x has a cause of its own, and this cause has a cause and so on. These causes may be called consecutive causes. Such causes form a chain and it is useful to distinguish the more immediate causes from the more remote ones. An example will make this clear.

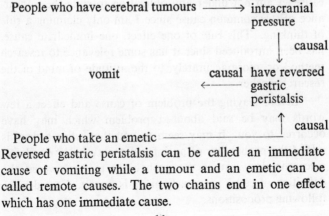

Reversed gastric peristalsis can be called an immediate cause of vomiting while a tumour and an emetic can be called remote causes. The two chains end in one effect which has one immediate cause.

11

Although we readily accept that an effect may have several remote causes, we have a sneaking feeling that it has only one immediate cause. This feeling or conviction encourages us to formulate the following rule although, it must be admitted, there is no empirical evidence or logical justification for the rule.

> Objects which are similar in one respect are similar in at least one other respect. Corollary: Objects which are different in one respect are different in at least one other respect.

At first you may deny this rule by saying, perhaps, that butter and yellow paint may both be yellow but that there is no other similarity. To this I would reply that there is a cause of yellowness and that this cause is common to both. And if you object that the cause of yellowness in butter and paint is different, I would reply that, as in the case of vomiting, there may be different remote causes but that this does not exclude the possibility of a common immediate cause. I am not under any obligation to state the appearance of this common cause since I am only claiming a rule of thinking. This rule of one effect, one immediate cause, has been introduced since it has some relevance to research method or, more accurately, to the attitude of mind of the research worker.

Before leaving the problem of cause and effect a few words may be said about a problem which may have occurred to you. It may seem to you that when a drug is *added* the probability of an inference may be *lowered* and since the drug causes the probability to be lowered the definition of cause previously given is wrong. Consider the following propositions.

who have pneumonia $\xrightarrow{\frac{2}{10}}$ die within two weeks.

People

and get penicillin $\xrightarrow{\frac{1}{10}}$ die within two weeks.

You will admit that, if dying within two weeks is an effect, penicillin can hardly be the cause. Indeed the definition of an effect is that it is an inference, the probability of which is raised when the cause is added and lowered when the cause is removed.

Explanations

You will frequently ask for, and be given, explanations and consequently they deserve some consideration. You may ask for an explanation of a property or for a correlative proposition. Here is an example.

Question: Why do people get headache?

Answer: People get headache because they have a cerebral tumour.

The explanation gives a cause of headache and derives from a correlative proposition as follows.

People with a cerebral tumour $\xrightarrow[\frac{8}{10}]{\text{causal}}$ have headache.

You will already appreciate that to establish cerebral tumour as a cause of headache, two propositions are required. It follows, therefore, that to give an explanation of headache, two correlative propositions must be known.

Here is another example.

Question: Why do people with cerebral tumour have headache?

Answer: People with cerebral tumour have headache because they have high intracranial pressure.

13

The explanation again gives a cause of headache but in this case the explanation derives from two propositions as follows.

$$\text{People with cerebral tumour} \xrightarrow[10]{\substack{\text{causal} \\ 6}} \substack{\text{have high} \\ \text{intracranal pressure.}}$$

$$\text{People with high intracranial pressure} \xrightarrow[10]{\substack{\text{causal} \\ 9}} \text{have headache.}$$

To establish tumour as a cause of high pressure two propositions are required and, similarly, to establish high intracranial pressure as a cause of headache two propositions are required. Consequently the explanation given above is based on four propositions.

You will now realise that explanations call for a considerable knowledge of correlative propositions. Furthermore, every effect has a large number of co-existent and consecutive causes and so innumerable causal propositions may be introduced.

Establishing properties as causes is tedious and sometimes impossible but many clinicians, rather than refuse on the ground of ignorance to give explanations, offer speculations, that is to say, explanations derived from speculative causal propositions. Unfortunately, the difficulty in verifying speculative explanations leads these clinicians to judge these explanations as true on the basis of the amount of conviction they arouse. In no field of human thought is *I think, therefore I am right* (perhaps it should be *I believe, therefore I am right**) more evident than in speculative explanations. It pervades all clinical medicine and especially psychiatry. A strong conviction is a good thing to have

---

* To give the dictum an air of authority it may be translated to *cogito, credo, ergo veritas est.*

if it drives you to verify your speculations. Otherwise it is a form of insanity.

Understanding

The word ' understanding ' has two meanings and this leads to some confusion. If you do not understand a word in empirical science then it may be concluded that either you do not know the appearance signified by the word or that you do not know the cause of the appearance signified by the word. Thus, if you say you do not understand coronary thrombosis, you may mean that you do not know what coronary thrombosis looks like pathologically or that you do not know the cause of coronary thrombosis. In the first case you are asking for a definition and in the second for an explanation.

You may, however, complicate the situation a little by claiming that you do not understand an explanation. Thus you may be told that atherosclerosis is the cause of coronary thrombosis and you may say that you do not understand how the former causes the latter. It should be evident to you by now that, when you ask how a cause produces an effect, you are really asking for an immediate cause to be put between the remote cause and its effect. It should also be evident to you that if, in our present example, you claim you do not know what causes atherosclerosis, you are embarking on an endless chain of causes or explanations.

Students often suppose that they must understand everything told to them. Certainly they must understand the meaning of words but they are undertaking a Herculean task if they insist on learning an explanation for every correlative proposition given to them by their teachers. Since an explanation is itself a correlative proposition, it follows that students are attempting to learn at least double the number of propositions required. This perhaps would be admirable if the students, as they nearly always do, would not give explanations priority over what is to be explained.

Similarities

If it is admitted that no two people are exactly alike in any respect, how can it be claimed that there are any similarities between people? The reason is that sometimes a difference of degree, time or place of a property can be ignored. A property is capable of analysis. Take, for example, a burn. This may occur at various times, in various places and be of various degrees of severity.

Let us suppose that a clinician sets out to make correlations between the delay in admitting a burn case to hospital and the response to a certain kind of treatment. He would first require to grade the response to treatment in some arbitrary way such as poor, moderate and good, and this division would have to be based on criteria accurately described by him. He would then divide his series of patients in terms of the interval of time between the burn and the admission to hospital. On examining his results he might possibly find that the patients who sustained their burns 24-48 hours before admission did poorly, that those who were burned 12-24 hours before admission did moderately well and that those who were burned within 12 hours of admission responded very well. He would now be in a position to say that a burn sustained 24-48 hours before admission was a point of similarity between certain patients on the basis that the inference in terms of the response to his particular treatment was the same. In the same way he could find similarities between his patients in terms of the site of the burn and its degree. To sum up, when the inference is the same, although the similarity is arbitrarily chosen, the variations in time, place and degree of the evidence can be ignored.

For a certain variation in a property to be ignored, however, not only must the inference be the same but also its probability. For example, the clinician may have shown that people with 24-48 hour burns have a probability of 3/10 of doing badly while the 12-24 hour burns have a probability of 1/10 of doing badly. The inference of the response to treatment is the same but the probability is different so that the variations in time before admission cannot be ignored. To ignore variations in time, place and degree of evidence, the inference must be the same and have the same probability.

It is pointless to argue about similarities and differences unless inferences are agreed upon. Imagine two doctors arguing about the severity of the burns of two patients. The first declares that they are of equal severity while the second declares that they are different. You will no doubt appreciate their annoyance when they discover that the first was inferring the danger to the patients if not transported to hospital by ambulance while the second was inferring the response to treatment after they had been admitted. With people who pursue the same kind of knowledge, arguments generally disappear when the inferences are agreed upon before the evidence is discussed.

Predictions

It is probable, from a biological point of view, that the purpose of thinking is to raise actions above the purely reflex level. In other words, we think in order to do. Thinking takes us from past and present situations to future ones. Furthermore, our own actions in the past and present are causes of future effects. It can, therefore, be said that we think in order to foresee the possible futures and we act in order to achieve the future we most desire.

In dealing with a patient our initial effort is to discover by a process of inference from evidence the various futures, including those brought about by different kinds of treatment, that lie in front of him and the probabilities of each. Otherwise we might find ourselves instituting potentially dangerous treatment in a patient who is almost certainly going to recover spontaneously, or trivial treatment in a patient who is likely to die. Needless to say the choice of futures properly lies with the patient but, should we choose it for him, we must do so on the assumption that it is the one he would choose himself if he was in possession of the relevant knowledge and in his right mind. When we are in doubt it is our obligation to discuss the matter with the patient or his relatives. We are not at liberty to put ourselves in the patient's place and choose a future accordingly, for the patient's values may be very different from our own. As in all other inter-personal relationships a little humility is desirable. Lastly, when we institute therapy in an effort to help a patient to gain his desired future, the only restriction imposed by our conscience and the State is that nothing we advise or do should have a greater probability of harming him than of helping him.

In making predictions it seems reasonable first to infer the type and site of pathology and then to infer the future state of the patient from this pathology with and without treatment. In doing so, however, we are making an assumption that our inference of pathology is necessarily correct. This we should not do, for assumptions have no part to play in correlative propositions. What is the alternative?

We constantly make use of propositions of the following kind, although we rarely have a precise knowledge of the numerical probabilities.

People with a slow hemiplegia $\xrightarrow{\frac{5}{10}}$ have a cerebral glioma.

People with a cerebral glioma $\xrightarrow{\frac{2}{10}}$ live for a year.

People with a slow hemiplegia $\xrightarrow{\frac{5 \times 2}{10 \times 10}}$ or $\xrightarrow{\frac{1}{10}}$ live for a year.

The first two propositions are products of research and the third necessarily follows from them. It would seem that, when we infer a glioma from the signs and then make predictions from it, we are making an inference from an inference. However, the slow hemiplegia is evidence while the glioma is not and the living for a year is inferred from the former and not from the latter. We have merely introduced the glioma in order to borrow the probabilities of the first two propositions for the purpose of calculating the probability of the third. We could perhaps say, since the glioma is not evidence and since we are not using it as an inference, that the term 'glioma' is being used merely as a symbol, and that what it is a symbol for is not important. It should be unnecessary to add that if pathology is verified by biopsy it becomes part of the evidence. You will notice that the calculated probability of the third proposition is less than that of the second and, for this reason, pathology should be verified if possible. It should also be unnecessary to add that, if a surgeon operates on a patient, the pathology is used as an inference and not merely as a means of calculating probabilities.

These remarks may explain why many clinicians who, in the course of their work, rarely see a pathological specimen, yet continue nevertheless to practise medicine efficiently. Furthermore, for such clinicians pathological terms often cease to signify histological and chemical appearances but stand rather as symbols for clinical evidence. Thus, instead of saying that a patient suffers from certain symptoms, they say merely that he is suffering from a certain kind of pathology. The pathological term is therefore used as an abbreviation. Apart from this it must be admitted that, since pathology is used as explanations and since everyone has a need for explanations, clinicians, who rarely see specimens, will continue to talk about pathology.

Causes are means of predicting future effects but predictions are often based on non-causal properties. For example, people who have a cerebral infarction and are deeply unconscious 12 hours after the onset will almost certainly die. You should therefore remember that in making predictions other properties are just as important as pathology. Indeed, you should realise that since pathology is usually no more than an inference from clinical evidence it is this evidence, as indicated above, which is used for predictions and not the pathology.

CHAPTER XX

THE LANGUAGE OF EMPIRICAL SCIENCE
(Continued)

Theoretical or hypothetical properties

Properties or appearances are limited by our sensory apparatus. For example, the hour hand of a watch moves so slowly and a bullet emerging from a gun moves so quickly that their movements are imperceptible. However, isolated positions of the hour hand and the bullet (in gun and target) can be seen and from these observations properties called 'moving hour hand' and 'moving bullet' are *constructed*. Since such constructed properties cannot be observed, although they have an appearance, they are called theoretical or hypothetical.

It may be wondered what is the purpose of constructing properties that cannot be seen. There is, of course, the satisfaction of connecting up isolated appearances into larger properties which contain them. The theoretical property, or theory for short, can be used as an explanation* of the isolated appearances. Thus the hour hand moves round the watch face and this is the explanation of the isolated appearances of the hand. The purpose of a theoretical property, however, is not to act as a satisfying explanation. Its purpose is to allow other properties to be deduced from it. You will notice that properties are deduced

---

* Explanation is used here in a new sense. Theoretical properties, being imperceptible, cannot be identified as causes and it follows that theoretical physics, for example, is concerned, not with causes, but only with predictions.

and this is another way of saying that, on the assumption that the theoretical property is correct, other properties *necessarily* follow from it.

It is necessary to say something about the verification of a theoretical property. Let us suppose that a house-fly buzzes round your head. On the basis of some observations you may construct a theoretical property that the fly moves in a circle of a certain radius at a constant specified speed. From this theory you could predict the time of arrival of the fly in front of your eyes. Now if the prediction is verified it does not prove your theory is correct for the fly may go round your head zig-zag, possibly pausing at your ears, and yet arrive at the specified place at the predicted time. A verified prediction, therefore, does not prove a theory. If, on the other hand, your prediction is found to be wrong then your theory is in part wrong. Thus one experiment may show a theory to be partly wrong but numerous experiments will never show it to be entirely correct.

When a theory gives rise to deductions which are shown to be wrong, the scientist, if he cares, may alter his theory to make allowance for the errors. Thus, by constructing theories, making deductions, putting them to the test and then modifying the theories on the basis of wrong deductions, theoretical scientific knowledge progresses. The more numerous the verified deductions from a theory the more reliable and acceptable it is. In evaluating a theory wrong deductions have to be balanced against correct ones but whether the theory should be retained or rejected is a problem for the individual scientist and no rules can be laid down. Always remember, however, that a theory, if it is to be called a theory, must lead to deductive inferences which, in principle at least, are observable.

Do not confuse theoretical properties (which cannot be seen) with properties which can be seen. For example, you may say that a penny is round but this statement is ambiguous. Firstly you may mean that the penny looks round and secondly you may mean that the penny is a perfect circle, the latter, of course, being an assumption. In the second case the roundness is theoretical and in the first it is not. From the theoretical property of roundness you may deduce the diameter of the penny but if you make no assumptions about roundness then nothing necessarily follows. To sum up, an inference is deductive when certainty connects the evidence and inference. Otherwise it is inductive. Obviously an inductive inference can only be based on observations of nature while deductive inferences can be made without reference to nature. It may also be added that you should not confuse a theoretical property with a speculative one. The former is a construction and the latter a mere product of the imagination. Most people make the terms 'theory' and 'hypothesis' synonymous with speculative correlative proposition but this is to be deplored.

A theoretical proposition may be taken as one which contains a theoretical property and a property deduced from it. Here is an example.

Cars which travel at a constant speed of 30 m.p.h. $\xrightarrow{\text{necessarily}}$ travel 15 miles in 30 minutes.

It is hoped that you will agree that a constant speed must always be an assumption.

There is a controversy among scientists about the nature of theoretical properties. Some believe that, although they are constructions, they nevertheless signify real appearances. Thus they would say that atoms are

23

theoretical but at the same time they do exist. Others think, however, that it is unimportant whether or not theoretical properties are real provided useful deductions can be made from them.

In routine clinical practice we rarely, if ever, employ theoretical properties.

At this point it may be helpful to recapitulate all the propositions which have been described.

Correlative propositions (verified and speculative, causal and non-causal). Inductive reasoning.

$$\text{Objects called } A \text{ which have } x \xrightarrow[m]{n} \text{ have } y$$
different appearances.

Definitive propositions.—

$$\text{Objects called } A \text{ which have } x \xrightarrow{\text{always}} \text{ have } y$$
same appearance or y is a part of the appearance of x.

Pseudo-correlative propositions.—Seductive reasoning.

$$\text{Objects called } A \text{ which have } x \xrightarrow[m]{n} \text{ have } y$$
y has no appearance or is very vague.

Theoretical propositions.—Deductive reasoning.

$$\text{Objects called } A \text{ which have } x \xrightarrow{\text{necessarily}} \text{ have } y$$
y is contained in x which is a construction and is assumed to be true.

Analogical thinking

Analogical thinking means thinking in terms of similarities. However, in common usage the meaning is more restricted. For example, comparing mice to men would be accepted as analogical thinking while comparing men to men would not. Indeed, it is difficult to see where the line is to be drawn between what is analogical and what is not. It is perhaps easier to speak of strong and weak analogies. A strong analogy consists of many similarities and few differences while a weak one consists of few similarities and many differences.

In the proposition

Objects called A which have x $\xrightarrow[m]{n}$ have y

the objects, apart from the similarities denoted by x and y, have similarities which bring them into the class called A. The grouping of similarities can now be shown

Objects called A which have x $\xrightarrow[m]{n}$ have y.

| Many or few similarities | several similarities. | one or few similarities |

The stronger the analogy the more general is the the proposition. A statement about a sample of common salt, for example, would be applicable to all samples for the analogy is nearly perfect. It is for this reason that in chemistry and physics one or two observations are sufficient for the formulation of a correlative proposition. In biology, on the other hand, analogies are not nearly so strong and large numbers of observations are required. As a corollary to the above statements it may be said that the weaker the analogy the less likely is a correlative proposition to be generally applicable.* Thus correlative propositions based on observations of mice may not be accurate, that is, the

---

* It is probably the number of differences, rather than the number of similarities, which determine the generality of a correlative proposition.

numerical probabilities may not be accurate, when applied to people.

Analogical thinking allows us to pass from one kind of object to another. Properties and correlations observed in one may be accepted as more or less verified, or less or more speculative, according to the strength or weakness respectively of the analogy when applied to the other. An advantage of analogical thinking is that, when faced with an unfamiliar situation, we can go to one which has some similarities to it and with which we are familiar. Having made observations on the familiar situation we can proceed to make useful speculations about the unfamiliar one.

Correlative propositions

A few remarks about correlative propositions have been left to the end since they refer to a rather difficult aspect of the subject.

Two correlative propositions can never contradict each other. Remember that a verified correlative proposition begins with the words *it has been observed by P* and when two people (or one person at different times) make a series of observations the circumstances may be different although this may not be known at the time the observations were made. Here are two abbreviated propositions.

$$\text{Water which is heated} \xrightarrow{\;\;\frac{\text{almost }10}{10}\;\;} \text{boils at } 100° \text{ C.}$$

$$\text{Water which is heated} \xrightarrow{\;\;\text{almost }0\;\;} \text{boils at } 100° \text{ C.}$$

It would seem that these propositions contradict each other and that only one can be a true statement of nature. However, investigation might show that the pressure under which the water of the second proposition was heated was

26

greater than that under which the water of the first proposition was heated. Thus the difference in the probability of two propositions may be accounted for by properties which are not included in the evidence. The only way in which exactly the same probability could be assured in two series of observations would be to ensure that the circumstances, which may be included as evidence, are identical. This, however, could never be ensured and even if it could, with the help of some supernatural power, the only conclusion would be that if things are unchanged then things are unchanged. This conclusion is simply a tautology and is scarcely interesting. You may now ask what your reaction should be to two propositions which are apparently contradictory. The answer is that you should believe both for the two observers formulating the propositions are probably quite honest. Of course, if you know that one of the observers is careless and that he often makes mistakes you would be justified in disregarding his propositions.

These remarks have considerable relevance to clinical medicine. Let us suppose that one clinician reports a recovery rate of 95 per cent. in the treatment of pneumonia with penicillin and another clinician reports only a 70 per cent. recovery rate. At first it would seem that one of them must be wrong but an enquiry may reveal that the first clinician observed only young patients while the second observed only old ones. You have already learned that the addition of properties to the evidence may change the probabilities of the inferences and consequently, when two propositions are contradictory, it is probable that one or both have a part of the evidence missing. Parts of evidence are omitted, of course, because the author is not aware that such parts influence the probabilities of his proposition. The difference between a good research worker and a bad one is that the former, unlike the latter, knows that a certain property changes the probabilities of a certain inference and he therefore includes this property in his statement of evidence. If he does not wish to include this property he makes sure that none of the patients he is talking about have it; or, if he cannot exclude it (for example, age), he makes sure that different degrees of the property are equally represented in his series of patients. For example, a clinician who wishes to make a statement of the incidence of lung cancer in coal miners would perhaps exclude cigarette smokers and, at the same time, he would arrange his series of subjects so that each age group contained the same numbers.

Perhaps the most awkward thing about correlative propositions is that one never follows necessarily from *one* other. If the slightest change is made in the evidence, as you are already aware, the probability may change in a completely unpredictable way. Worse still, a proposition true at this moment is not necessarily true one moment from now. Once a set of observations have been made the circumstances under which they were made may immediately change; at least we cannot guarantee that they will not and consequently when a second set of observations is made the probability may have altered. It would seem, therefore, that we cannot progress *logically* from one correlative proposition to another, nor can we be sure that a correlative proposition will remain valid after the passage of time. It is fortunate, with regard to the latter difficulty, that circumstances do not change a great deal and *experience* shows that a correlative proposition made today will be valid tomorrow. This may perhaps be clearer in the form of a correlative proposition.

Propositions which have a certain probability based on observations made today	$\xrightarrow{\frac{9}{10}}$	will have the same probability based on observations made tomorrow.

The probability of this proposition is high when we are talking about dead matter but not very high when we are talking about living things.

Conclusion

It is hoped that the remarks given under the heading of The Language of Empirical Science will not be interpreted as instructions in methods of thinking. On the contrary, they consist only of an analysis of language and what relevance they have to thinking lies only in the fact that thinking is sometimes performed by means of words. It is possible, if not probable, that your reading of these chapters has provoked a feeling of disappointment that, since one correlative proposition never follows necessarily from another, no great reasoning power is required in empirical science. If this is so, you should be consoled by the thought that your ideas of reasoning have been rather vague and based largely on the thought processes which underlie the construction of theoretical properties and the so-called natural laws. Admittedly, the synthesis of observations into a theory or natural law (a natural law is simply a theory which has led to many verified deductions) requires a high level of intelligence but this is not necessarily of a higher order than that required for the formulation of speculative correlative propositions, for their verification by observation and for the identification of properties as causes.

Perhaps the analysis of language will help you to read medical articles more critically. Being critical, however, does not mean being incredulous or destructive. It means being at first analytical and this in turn means finding out the kinds of propositions authors use, the evidence they describe in terms of x and y (inferences are not allowed in statements of research results), the precision of definition of their terms, the precision of the probabilities and the methods they employ in identifying causes. Many authors, unfortunately, mix together correlative, definitive and pseudo-correlative propositions and your analysis may be tedious and irritating but once completed you will find it surprisingly easy to assess, for doctors in general and yourself in particular, the value of what you read. Nearly always the evidence which you will identify as y is of a sort which is of little or no interest to the practising doctor and the evidence you will identify as x is of a sort which the practising doctor is quite unable to observe for want of suitable equipment. Consequently, the material you may wish to memorise can be readily reduced to manageable proportions.

CHAPTER XXI

CLINICAL EVIDENCE AND INFERENCES

Changing probabilities

In Volume I it was shown that, by building up evidence, the probabilities of inferences could be raised or lowered. Clinical evidence consists largely of symptoms, signs and the results of special investigation, but other observations may be included. The age and sex of the patient, the family history and occupational and social environment may all be important. In neurology the age and family history are of special significance. Age is of particular importance, for most neurological diseases occur within fairly well defined age limits.

The choice of inferences

It is necessary to say something about the initial inferences which are made from the first piece of evidence, that is, the patient's complaint. When a patient complains of a cough, for example, we may infer bronchitis, pulmonary tuberculosis, pneumonia, bronchial carcinoma and so on. The number of possible inferences is, of course, very large and for this reason it is advisable to put them in order in terms of their probabilities, putting the one with the highest probability at the top of the list and the one with the lowest at the bottom. To put inferences in order of probability, however, requires a knowledge of the incidence of disease in the community in which you find yourself. Unfortunately, your teachers will make little reference to the incidence of disease and indeed, if your hospital training is of the usual kind, you will get your inferences in the wrong order since hospital doctors are apt to specialise in rare diseases rather than common ones. If you are aware of this you will at least go into medical practice knowing that you have still to learn the proper order of inferences from the various complaints that you will hear.

When you are making your first inferences from a patient's complaint you have to decide how far down you should go in the scale of probabilities towards the rare diseases. The decision should rest on the amount of experience you have accumulated. Thus, if you are inexperienced, you should not venture beyond the common conditions whereas, if you have a wide experience, you may wander into the realm of rare diseases. Remember that if you never diagnose rare diseases you will rarely be wrong whereas, if you frequently diagnose rare diseases, you will frequently be wrong.

Repeated examinations

So far no effort has been made to quantify clinical signs, for the quantity has no diagnostic value with regard to the site of the lesion. However, when you are able to examine a patient on several occasions, the changing quantity of signs enables you to add to the sign-time graph which you have already constructed on the basis of the history. Unfortunately, it is difficult to measure most signs with any precision and you must be satisfied with rough measurements. In the early stages of your professional life you must become expert at detecting signs before you try estimating their degree and, even when you start to estimate degree, you must be content with only a few gradations. Three grades which may be called slight, moderate and gross are all that is required, although it is a matter of personal choice how this gradation is to be put into practice. You will find, no doubt, that you will fall into a system of your own and, although you may have difficulty in describing the grades to others, you will find them reliable and useful in your own work.

Organic lesion and functional disorder

The term 'organic lesion' is commonly used by clinicians and yet you would have difficulty in finding a clinician who would offer a fairly precise definition. Clearly, organic lesion signifies a type of abnormal property but which type is the question. In an effort to find the common medical usage of the term, properties have been divided into several types in Figure 53. This classification has nothing to do with making inferences and is concerned only with definitions. Before examining this classification we must take a look at the word 'lesion'. A lay dictionary defines it as injury or damage but clinicians make the term stand for much more than this. Thus, an abscess would be called a lesion although it consists of many histological appearances apart from damaged tissue. Similarly a neoplasm, sometimes called a space-occupying lesion, consists

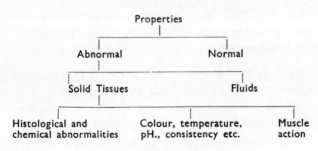

FIG. 53
A Classification of Properties.

33

of tumour cells which are not damaged cells in the ordinary sense. We are, therefore, justified in assuming that a lesion is no more nor less than an abnormal histological appearance. If you now look at the classification you will see that abnormal properties are divided into those relevant to solid tissues and fluids. The reason for this is that an abnormal histological appearance of blood and cerebrospinal fluid would not be called a lesion. Properties of solid tissues are further divided, for a raised temperature of the skin would not be called a lesion of the skin; also the contraction of an artery, due to action of its muscle coats, would not be called a lesion of the artery. We may now reach the conclusion that an organic lesion, according to common usage, is a histological abnormality of solid tissue. Presumably the term ' organic lesion ' could only be applied on the basis of naked-eye appearances if histological abnormalities could be inferred with something approaching certainty.

It seems rather absurd to draw a distinction between solids and fluids in the definition of organic lesion. Furthermore, since staining reactions are chemical reactions, it would be unwise to draw a distinction between histological and chemical abnormalities. Accordingly the following definition is suggested.

> An organic lesion is a histological or chemical abnormality.

We have, of course, now pushed ourselves into the curious position of calling albuminuria an organic lesion of urine but this is not important in view of what is to be gained from a precise definition of organic lesion.

The terms ' physical lesion ' and ' organic lesion ' are synonymous but the word ' physical ' alone is not synonymous with either. Thus, to say that all pain has a physical cause is not equivalent to saying that all pains are caused by an organic lesion, unless, of course, the latter statement is speculative. It is perhaps obvious that experience reveals that only some pains are caused by organic lesions, although experience with new microscopic and chemical techniques may increase the number of pains caused by organic lesions. It is worth noting at this point that any property may be a cause, whether or not it may be called an organic lesion.

A series of propositions may be written as follows.

People with convulsions $\xrightarrow{\frac{1}{1,000}}$ have a cerebral tumour.

People with convulsions $\xrightarrow{\frac{1}{500}}$ have a cerebral scar.

People with convulsions $\xrightarrow{\frac{1}{10,000}}$ have hypoglycaemia.
etc.   etc.

We may now summarise these propositions by the following statement.

People with convulsions $\xrightarrow{\frac{1}{100}}$ have cerebral organic lesions.

We may proceed to speculate that all convulsions are caused by a cerebral abnormality or disorder and on this basis we may formulate the following proposition.

People with convulsions $\xrightarrow{\frac{99}{100}}$ have a cerebral functional disorder.

You will notice that the new numerical probability is obtained by subtracting the probability of an organic lesion from one. You must realise that the term 'cerebral functional disorder' does not signify an appearance and that the above proposition is pseudo-correlative. All that we mean by the proposition is that we think the cerebrum is a

35

good place to look for as yet undiscovered causes of convulsions. In other words, we are speculating about the site of unknown abnormal properties.

It is apparent that an organic sign is a piece of evidence which allows a high probability inference of an organic lesion while a functional sign is a piece of evidence which allows only a low probability inference of an organic lesion. You should remember that the term ' functional disorder ' is meaningless unless an organ or body part is specified.

Sometimes a part of the body seems to be an almost necessary link in a certain causal chain. For example, an increased flow of saliva seems certainly to be due to the salivary glands. Provided no organic lesion is found in the glands we may say, without apparently speculating, that an increased flow of saliva is due to a functional disorder of the salivary glands. All we are saying, of course, is that the glands are a cause and the saliva is an effect. The statement that a certain body part seems to be a necessary link in a certain causal chain is of no value in routine clinical medicine unless we are prepared to remove the part in an effort to cure the effect. In other words, to get rid of an unknown abnormal property* we have no alternative to removing the part where the property is, if, for the moment, you will excuse this kind of language.

It is unfortunate that many clinicians make the terms ' functional ' and ' psychogenic ' synonymous. Thus, to many clinicians, the statement that convulsions are a functional disorder means that they are caused by the mind. Of course we are very careless in our use of language when we say that convulsions are a functional disorder for what

---

* It would appear to be necessarily true that an abnormal property, considered as an effect, must have an abnormal property as a cause. For example, an abnormally large flow of saliva must be caused by an abnormal property of the salivary glands.

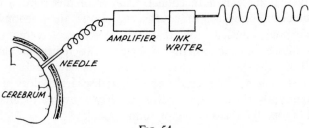

FIG. 54
The Recording of Brain Waves.

we really mean is that convulsions, with a high probability, are related (at least, so we speculate) to a functional disorder of the cerebrum; and what we really mean by this is that convulsions allow only a low probability inference of a cerebral organic lesion although we nevertheless speculate that the cerebrum is a cause of all convulsions. The confusion engendered by the terms 'functional' and 'psychogenic' would certainly be avoided if it was agreed that the former only means the absence of an organic lesion without at the same time implying that the mind is in any way involved.

Before leaving this difficult subject a few words must be said about electricity. In Figure 54 a wire, insulated except at its tip, is shown implanted in a cerebrum. The wire is led to an amplifier which is linked with a pen-writer. The waves written on the paper by the pen-writer constitute evidence. What is the inference? Clearly something is happening at the tip of the needle and we may safely conclude that the cerebrum at the tip of the needle is a link in a causal chain which has the waves as an effect. Examination of this piece of cerebrum may reveal organic lesions or some other kind of physical property but in many instances nothing unusual may be found. We may therefore

37

say that there is a functional disorder of this portion of cerebrum provided, of course, the waves are abnormal. We may, indeed, say that this portion of cerebrum is discharging abnormally as long as we remember that all we are saying is that it appears to be a link in a causal chain. The term ' abnormal discharge ' does not signify a verified or speculative property or even a theoretical property. It is a name for nothing.

CHAPTER XXII

CEREBRAL SEGMENTAL SIGNS

YOU will remember that two long tracts end in the cerebrum, namely the pyramidal tracts and the posterior columns. It will be suggested later that the optic radiations should be considered as long tracts. We have now to deal with the rest of the cerebrum, the parts which may be called cerebral segments. The signs now to be described are, therefore, of a segmental type, that is, signs from which cerebral segmental lesions may be inferred.

Unfortunately a difficulty arises in dealing with the cerebrum. Normal cerebral activity depends a great deal on other organs. Thus, a failure of the heart to send blood to the cerebrum may cause the latter to perform inefficiently. It is now apparent that when we elicit a cerebral segmental sign we have the problem of deciding whether to rest content with an inference of an immediate cause in the cerebrum or whether to feel obliged to make an inference of a remote cause in another organ. For example, in the case of a patient who has fainted, should we rest content with an inference of cerebral anoxia or should we push on and try to find a remote cause such as heart block? In practice, when we are thinking in terms of possible therapy, the following rules are helpful.

1. When the immediate cause of a symptom or sign is a chemical abnormality of the cerebrum (*e.g.* anoxia) it is advisable to search thoroughly for a remote cause elsewhere.

CEREBRAL SEGMENTAL SIGNS

PSYCHOLOGICAL

Mood disorder   Behaviour disorder   Perceptual disorder   Thought disorder
                                           (hallucinations)

Personality disorder

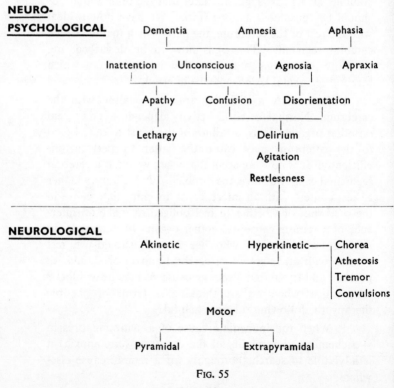

**NEURO-
PSYCHOLOGICAL**

NEUROLOGICAL

FIG. 55

2. When the immediate cause of a symptom or sign is a histological abnormality of the cerebrum there is no need to look elsewhere for a cause except when the immediate cause is secondary tumour or abscess. There are several other exceptions.

In cerebral disorders it is convenient to think of evidence in three compartments (Fig. 55) called neurological, neuro-psychological and psychological.

Neurological evidence

Previously we have considered motor disorders in terms of weakness and changes in muscle tone. In the present context we will confine ourselves to movement considered quantitatively. The quantity of motor activity exhibited by a patient may be greater or less than normal. The amount of motor activity exhibited by normal people, of course, varies a great deal but at the moment we are thinking of pathological extremes. If you have a fondness for scientific terminology you can call the extremes akinetic and hyperkinetic.

Excessive movements are of various types.

1. Chorea consists of short, sharp, rapid movements usually of small excursion. Hemiballismus is a variation in which the limbs make considerable movements.

2. Athetosis consists of slow sinuous movements often of considerable amplitude. The movements may occur in the neck and trunk as well as the limbs and may then be called torsion spasms.

3. Tremor consists of rhythmic to and from movements and, when it has a neurological cause, it is slow and coarse. The movements usually have a small amplitude but occasionally are gross.

41

The common characterstics of the three types of movements are as follows.

1. They are involuntary, by which is meant that the patient is powerless to stop them.

2. They are continuous while the patient is awake and absent in sleep. This statement will later be modified in the case of tremor.

3. They are purposeless, that is, the movements are not directed towards any desired end.

4. They are aggravated by excitement and embarrassment.

There is another type of excessive movement called a convulsion but this deserves special mention in a later chapter.

Apart from the excessive movements so far described the patient may exhibit general restlessness, the more severe degree of which may be called agitation. Restless movements may be entirely purposeful, as for example when a patient constantly walks backwards and forwards, semi-purposeful or non-purposeful. Incessant talking may be considered a kind of restlessness.

Neuro-psychological evidence

For convenience the neuro-psychological functions of the cerebrum can be put under seven headings as follows.

Attention.	Memory.
Consciousness.	Language function.
Intelligence.	Spatial perception.
Purposeful movement.	

It is necessary, however, to stop for a moment and decide what we mean by function in this connection. Certainly consciousness is a function or effect of the cerebrum for without the cerebrum there is no consciousness. Unfortunately, if we assume that consciousness is a normal function of the cerebrum, we are apt to suppose that from consciousness we can assume a normal cerebrum. This supposition, however, is entirely wrong for a patient may be conscious and yet have a very abnormal cerebrum. It is nevertheless true that since normal people are conscious and have a normal cerebrum, we are justified in inferring a normal cerebrum with a high probability from consciousness but this correlation is of no clinical value.

The way out of the difficulty provoked by the use of the word 'consciousness' is to drop the word altogether and use instead another property called 'unconsciousness'. The advantage is that from unconsciousness an abnormal cerebrum can be inferred with a high probability and this clearly has great clinical importance.

The remarks made about consciousness are equally applicable to attention, intelligence and so on. We have thus to substitute seven other properties and these are as follows.

Inattention.	Amnesia.
Unconsciousness.	Aphasia.
Dementia.	Spatial agnosia.

Apraxia.

It should be emphasised that the terms 'inattention', 'unconsciousness' and so on signify properties. To be more explicit, they are ways in which a patient behaves in a situation which you as an examiner have created. The terms, or rather their synonyms, may, of course, be used by the patient's relatives and friends, but again they signify the behaviour of the patient in certain circumstances. The great difficulty which arises is that the terms may overlap in meaning, that is to say, one kind of behaviour may allow two terms to be applied. From the point of view of accuracy of description this is disappointing but the consolation is that each kind of behaviour is a cerebral segmental sign from which a cerebral lesion may be inferred. The precise separation of the patient's behaviour in types is, therefore, not very important.

Inattention

Like so many clinical words the word ' inattention ' has two meanings. While being interviewed by you the patient may exhibit inattention in the sense that he readily directs his attention from you to other events in the ward. In short, he is easily distracted and it could almost be said that he has too much attention since anything catches his eye. According to the meaning of the word ' inattention ' which we are going to adopt this sort of behaviour would not be called inattentive. For our present purpose it is best to restrict the meaning of the word to little or no attention for anything. The patient not only does not attend to you but apparently does not attend to anything, presumably not even his own thoughts. There are various grades of inattention which are probably best defined by the time during which the patient's attention can be held. For example, a patient whose attention lapses after a moment or two could be said to be moderately inattentive while a patient whose attention cannot be held even for a moment could be said to be very or completely inattentive.

Unconsciousness

Unconsciousness means unresponsiveness. Several levels can be differentiated on the basis of the stimulus which fails to provoke a response on the part of the patient.

1. Fails to respond to any stimulus.

2. (*a*) Responds only to pain.

(*b*) Responds (that is, directs attention) to noises, including the examiner's voice.

3. Responds to simple commands by obeying them. Such commands are: open your eyes, shut your eyes, put your tongue out, hold your hand up and so on. When the patient is aphasic he responds to gestures or performs, spontaneously, simple acts such as rubbing the eyes, adjusting the blankets or clothing and so on.

4. Responds to complex commands by obeying them. Such commands are used in routine neurological examination. When the patient is aphasic he performs, spontaneously, complex acts such as feeding and dressing.

These levels seem quite straightforward but there are some difficulties.

1. It may be asked in what way level 4 differs from the consciousness of a normal person. The answer is that there is no difference. This would seem to commit us to the absurdity of saying that a normal person has a level 4 unconsciousness but this strangely enough should not disturb us since inferences of cerebral abnormalities will not be inferred from this level.

2. It would seem that a totally inattentive patient would present the same appearance as a patient with unconscious level 1 or 2. The distinction to be drawn, however, is that the inattentive patient will still continue to perform complex acts and this may be taken as a measure of his responsiveness to his environment. If it is objected that responsiveness to the environment implies attentiveness it must be admitted that total inattention and unconscious level 1 are synonymous.

3. It may be asked how unconscious levels are to be distinguished from the appearance of a person intentionally assuming these modes of behaviour. The answer is that on the basis of definitions so far given no distinction can be drawn.

4. The distinction between sleep and unconscious level 1 seems at first difficult. It is obvious, however, that a sleeping patient may be roused while the unconscious patient who responds perhaps to pain will not be raised to higher levels. It is perhaps worth adding that no distinction can be drawn between a patient who is sleeping and a patient who is assuming sleep.

Dementia

It is advisable, in the present context, to rob intelligence of its mysticism and define it as a mode of behaviour. In scientific terms it would be defined as a specific mode of behaviour in certain test situations.

The testing of intelligence is a highly specialised pursuit quite outside the scope of the average clinician and the reason for this is that the psychologist and the clinician are trying to do different things. When a psychologist measures a subject's I.Q. he is gathering evidence from which the subject's future behaviour in circumstances, not immediately relevant to his everyday life, can be predicted. Thus when a boy's I.Q. is measured a prediction can be made about his behaviour and performance in future environments and occupations. Perhaps it should be stated at this point that behaviour, performance and appearance are all synonymous in the present context. The clinician, on the other hand, measures intelligence since from the results he can infer cerebral disease and the patient's future performance in his ordinary pursuits. Furthermore, repeated tests of intelligence may allow the clinician to elaborate a sign-time graph from which he may infer the type of cerebral pathology.

Although clinicians rarely practise formal intelligence testing they nevertheless become fairly expert in the rough assessment of intelligence. The manner in which a patient conducts himself during an interview, the history he gives and the grasp of the part he has to play in a physical examination can all be described in terms of intelligent or unintelligent behaviour. In the assessment of such behaviour it is not so much the patient's accuracy that matters but his ability to cope with the novel problem of a medical examination. Of course the patient's abilty to cope will be influenced by inattention, unconsciousness and aphasia but, when such signs are present, a measurement of dementia is not important diagnostically since cerebral disease can already be inferred with a high probability.

It is important that you should have at least a nodding acquaintance with intelligence testing and the following quick and superficial analysis may serve this purpose.

Intelligence tests can be divided into two groups which may be called verbal and non-verbal. In the first the patient's ability to use symbols is examined and in the second his ability to make comparisons. The division between the two kinds of tests, however, is not clear-cut for verbal instructions are used in non-verbal tests and the ability to compare underlies some verbal tests.

Verbal tests.—There are a variety of such tests, an important one being the vocabulary test. In this the patient is asked to give simple definitions of words which range from the easy to the difficult. This is a useful test for the results allow an assessment of the patient's educational level and also because it is claimed that in a dementia the vocabulary is the last of the intelligence test performances to suffer. The performance in the vocabulary test can therefore be used as a base line for the other tests. In another test the patient is asked to provide words of similar and opposite meaning to a selection of given words. Several other tests may be enumerated.

1. The patient has to rearrange the jumbled letters of words and the jumbled words of sentences.

2. The patient has to complete words and sentences from which parts are missing.

3. The patient has to analyse a complex order. For example, I might ask you to underline the letter which is placed before the first a after the second e in this sentence.

4. The patient has to interpret stories and proverbs.

Non-verbal tests.—Most of these tests are designed to measure the patient's ability to observe and to detect similarities and differences. A few common tests will be enumerated.

1. Comparison of individuals. The usual test is to confront the patient with a series of pictures all of which are similar except one which he has to detect. A variation of this is one in which the patient has to supply the missing part of a pattern from several patterns which are all different. In another test the patient is shown a number of objects and asked to sort them into groups on the basis of similarities. Usually the objects can be sorted using shape or colour as the point of similarity. Lastly, the patient may be asked to point out a similarity between pairs of objects given verbally such as apple and orange, and dog and cat.

2. Comparison of pairs. In testing comparisons of this kind, words, numbers or objects may be used, the last generally in the form of pictures. In performing these tests

the patient has to detect a property of each pair which is similar in all pairs. The property of a pair may be a difference or similarity between its individuals or a relationship between them. Here are three examples.

> Dog is to puppy as cat is to …?…
> Doctor is to hospital as teacher is to …?…
> 2   4   6   8 ……… add the next two terms.

3. Classification. The sorting test mentioned above could be put in this category. Usually, however, the patient is given a list of nouns and asked to put into groups or classes the objects they signify. Here is an example.

> Put into classes the following people.
> Surgeon. School teacher. Singer. Doctor.
> Office worker. Dancer. Latin master. General
> practitioner. Clown. Head master. Typist.
> Accountant.

4. Deduction. There is a large variety of tests which measure the patient's ability to make deductive inferences. In these tests the word deduction is correctly used in that one statement necessarily follows from another but in the tests the deductions are based on numbers or definitions rather than on theoretical properties. Tests with numbers consist of simple arithmetical problems. A favourite one is the 100-7 test in which the patient subtracts 7 from 100 and then 7 from the remainder and so on. Tests without numbers are best shown by means of an example with which you are no doubt familiar.

> A man looking at a portrait declares that he
> has no brothers and that the father of the
> man portrayed is his father's son. Who is the
> man in the picture?

The difficulty in such problems lies largely in the complexity of the instructions.

Conclusions.—If you find intelligence testing interesting you should refer to one of the many publications in this field. In routine practice, however, you will almost certainly have to rely on an assessment of the patient's intelligence based on his behaviour during an ordinary medical examination. Dementia, of course, would only be diagnosed if your assessment of the patient's intelligence fell below the level you expected on the basis of his scholastic career and his occupation. Should you want to confirm this assessment with some specialised tests you should confine yourself to the vocabulary test, the interpretation of stories and proverbs and simple mathematical problems. Questions on general knowledge, a test commonly practised by clinicians, is more a test of memory than of intelligence.

Amnesia

A fairly good estimation of the patient's memory can be made during the history-taking when he gives an account of previous illnesses and the development of present symptoms. There are numerous tests of a more specialised kind but only a few will now be enumerated.

1. The patient is asked to give the dates of various national and international events which have occurred during his lifetime. Alternatively, he can be asked to name important people connected with these events.

2. A standard sentence is read to the patient and he is then asked to repeat it. Should he fail to do so accurately the sentence is read again and such repetitions may be continued until the patient successfully reproduces it. The sentences are designed in such a way that a normal subject requires two or three attempts. It is not the patient's failure

which indicates amnesia so much as the failure to improve as the sentence is repeated to him. Here is an example of this kind of test sentence.

> The old man was wearing a dark blue suit,
> shiny and stained with constant use, and on
> his feet were tattered shoes which did little to
> protect their owner from the cold and rain.

3. The patient is asked to repeat a series of digits read to him. The series starts with two digits and this number is progressively increased. Normal subjects can memorise about seven digits.

4. The patient is asked to draw from memory simple designs which he has been allowed to examine for about a minute. You will see later that tests of spatial memory are included in tests of spatial agnosia.

The patient's performance in these tests may of course be influenced by inattention, unconsciousness and aphasia. On the whole, memory tests are more valuable clinically than intelligence tests. The reason probably is that there is not much difference between normal people in their memory test performance while there is considerable difference in their intelligence test performance. A patient whose memory test performance, therefore, is poor, can be considered to have a cerebral lesion with a high probability.

Aphasia

A patient is said to be aphasic when he cannot use symbols whether verbal, mathematical or musical. There are all grades of impairment in the use of symbols and it is customary to use the term ' aphasia ' to signify a severe impairment and ' dysphasia ' to signify a slight or moderate impairment. Little is to be gained by using these two words since they are given no precise definition. It is best to use aphasia to cover all grades and to specify the grade with other words such as slight, moderate and severe.

It is traditional to divide aphasia into different kinds but this is futile for the inference from each type, clinically at least, is the same. A common distinction which is made is between expressive and receptive aphasia, terms which are self-explanatory, and these may be retained for they signify disabilities which have a bearing on the patient's everyday life.

It is sufficient in routine clinical practice to assess the patient's ability to speak and to understand the spoken word. The history-taking and examination reveal all but the slightest grades of aphasia. The patient may have difficulty in answering your questions and it will be apparent to you that:

> He makes noises which, at most, are reminiscent of words (jargon aphasia),
> *or* his grammar is confused,
> *or* he sometimes cannot find a word which is appropriate to his answers or that he uses the wrong word.

On the other hand, the patient may not understand your questions and commands (receptive aphasia) but since this receptive failure is nearly always accompanied by an expressive failure it is not of importance diagnostically.

Should you decide to make a special search for aphasia there are two things that you may do.

1. You may ask the patient to name a series of about 20 common objects, such as a watch, pencil, button, pin and so on, which are shown to him.

2. You may engage the patient in conversation as distinct from a question and answer relationship, encourage-

ing him to speak spontaneously on various familiar and unfamiliar topics. Unfortunately your clinical training does not include practice in conversation with patients on non-medical subjects and at first you will feel inept. Should a conversion lag remind yourself that few people can resist talking about themselves and their ideas to someone who is apparently interested.

It may be mentioned in conclusion that it is absurd to talk about evidence of aphasia. Aphasia is evidence.

Spatial agnosia* (Achorognosia)

It has been previously said that a diminution of somatic spatial feeling may be caused by a lesion anywhere from the sensory endings in skin, joints, muscles and tendons and the parietal lobes. We have now to consider disorders of spatial thinking for these are a product of lesions confined to the parietal lobes. Just what we mean by thinking in this connection is rather vague. The distinction between sensation and perception, too, is somewhat blurred but clinically this is not important. We may take it that anything other than a raising of spatial feeling thresholds (visual and somatic) is a segmental cerebral sign.

The space which we feel is exterior to our sensory surfaces but this is a tautology, for space and outsideness are synonymous. We have no feeling of space interior to our sensory surfaces and this you will confirm by trying to feel the space inside your skull. Of course, we can see the space of our hand, for example, and we can feel its space with the other hand but this hand space is clearly external to the sensory surfaces of the eye and of the other hand. By exploring our body with eyes and hands we are therefore able to have thoughts about ourselves as an object.

* Other types of agnosia are described but they are of little importance clinically.

We are able, as it is sometimes said, to have an image of our body.

Apart from this body image, however, we have certain feelings which are not in themselves spatial. Should we hold an arm in the air we may say that we feel our arm maintaining a posture. This feeling of posture amounts to a spatial feeling but what do we mean when we say that we *feel* our arm? This problem, too, is made more acute by the fact that this feeling of an arm would persist even if the arm were amputated. Clearly the feeling has no immediate causal relation with the nerves of the arm. The feeling of a limb which persists after amputation is often referred to as a phantom although calling it a name does not solve our present problem. Reflection on this problem forces us to the conclusion that it is nonsensical to ask what we mean when we say we feel our arm since there is no way of defining any feeling. Nevertheless to pose the problem draws our attention to those feelings which do not immediately depend on peripheral sensory impulses. Most clinicians use body image and body feeling (in its present context) as synonymous terms although, as has been indicated, the former refers to the body viewed objectively and the latter to it viewed subjectively. For the present the term ' body image ' will be taken to include body feeling.

It has been necessary to introduce this rather muddled topic of body image for patients may experience distortions of the image or even its loss. Thus a hand, for example, may seem to the patient to have grown in size or diminished, or he may lose his image of one side of his body.*

---

* An occasional patient, without loss of body image, will deny weakness on his hemiplegic side. The inconsistency between his statement and performance apparently escapes him.

The latter defect, as you can imagine, leads to difficulty in dressing.

Space itself presents problems which are analogous to those of body image and body feeling. Thus a man who is blinded continues to be aware of dark space so that dark space could be called a phantom. Patients, too, may experience distortions of space and one side of space may be lost. Another feature common to body image and space is that of orientation, by which we mean the distinction between right and left, up and down, and near and far. As a result of a parietal lobe lesion a patient may not be able to make these distinctions and, consequently, he may become lost even in familiar surroundings and he may have the difficulty in dressing already mentioned.

Leaving aside body image and spatial orientation, there are some simpler defects of spatial thinking which consist of an inability to make spatial comparisons and to observe spatial similarities and differences. This inability, furthermore, may be complicated by a spatial memory defect. As a result the patient may not be able to recognise objects, visually or tactually, and this is not surprising when it is remembered that objects all have a spatial property.

These defects of spatial thinking which have been described may be demonstrated by suitable tests and several will now be enumerated.

1. The patient is asked to indicate his right and left hands.

2. He is asked to identify objects shown to him, visually and tactually. Due allowance must, of course, be made for aphasia if this is present.

3. He is asked to indicate on a piece of paper, placed in front of him, the edge which is nearest and the one

which is furthest. He may also be asked to indicate right and left.

4. He is asked to bisect a line drawn on the paper or to indicate the centre of a circle.

5. He is asked to copy simple designs directly and from memory.

6. He is asked to draw from memory a simple object such as a chair.

7. He is asked to draw a clock face and to draw the hands indicating a specified time.

8. He is asked to draw a simple plan of the living room of his house.

9. He is asked to copy a simple design with matches.

10. He is asked to copy with coloured blocks (Koh's blocks) a design which is shown to him.

11. He is asked to dress.

12. He is taken from his ward to another part of the hospital and asked to make his own way back.

This seems a formidable list but, of course, the tests are only pursued to the point where you have gathered convincing evidence.

There is another cerebral segmental sensory sign which must be mentioned since this is different from those described above. A normal person who is touched or pricked on both hands simultaneously is aware of the two sensations. A patient, however, who has a parietal lobe lesion, may not have two sensations although he may feel a touch or a pin-prick on either hand when the stimulation is not simultaneous. It is sometimes said that the feeling in the affected hand, that is the hand opposite to the affected parietal lobe, is extinguished by the feeling in the normal hand. This statement, it should be noted, is descriptive of the result of bilateral simultaneous stimulation rather than an explanation of the result. This test of sensory extinction is a good one for it may be the only one to reveal an abnormality.

It is hoped that you will have the opportunity of seeing a patient with a spatial agnosia for a demonstration of signs will help to elucidate what is otherwise a difficult subject.

Apraxia

Apraxia is the motor counterpart of achorognosia and means an inability to perform purposeful movements. Patients who have muscular weakness, cerebellar inco-ordination, achoraesthesia or achorognosia may also have difficulty in such movements and the term ' apraxia ' should therefore only be used when such signs are absent.

The neuro-psychological compartment contains several other terms such as apathy, confusion and so on. These terms are used a good deal by clinicians but, unfortunately, they do not have precise definitions. In the present context they have been given a distinct neurological bias and you will see in Figure 55 that they are considered to be derived from combinations of other terms. The term ' delirium ' includes confusion, disorientation and agitation but may also include terms from the psychological compartment under the headings of perceptual and thought disorders. Lastly, it may be added that urinary and faecal incontinence, to which the patient is indifferent, may be caused by a cerebral lesion.

Psychological evidence

The disorders of behaviour, emotion, thought and perception are many and varied and call for additional terminology. This terminology you will learn in psychiatry

CLINICAL AND LAY TERMINOLOGY

Neurological Terminology	Lay Terminology	Psychiatric Terminology
Dementia	Mental slowness	Disorders of thought
Amnesia	Failure of judgment	and behaviour
Agnosia	Inefficiency	
	Confusion	
	Deterioration of social and moral behaviour	
	Lack of Initiative	
	Restlessness	
	Disorientation	
Inattention	Failure of concentration	Disorders of emotion
	Apathy	(depression, shallowness
	Irritability	and elation)
	Agitation	
Unconsciousness	Delirium	Disorders of perception
	Confusion	(hallucinations and illusions)

FIG. 56

and if you have not already done so you should now read descriptions of manic-depressive psychosis and schizophrenia. As you do this you should add some of the terms to Figure 56 under the heading Psychiatric Terminology. The disorders signified by these terms may be collectively covered by the term ' psychosis '.

You will see from Figure 56 that the terminology relating to disorders of cerebral function is extensive and this accounts for a good deal of the difficulty experienced by the student when he is studying this part of neurology. Under the heading Neurological Terminology are the various terms which have already been described. However, there is a large list of terms used by the lay public (and often by clinicians) and such terms are of great use in history-taking. Unfortunately these terms signify disorders which may be covered by neurological terminology on the one hand or by psychiatric terminology on the other. Nevertheless it is very important to keep a clear distinction between neuro-psychological and psychological signs for the inferences from each are different as will be revealed in a later chapter.

The term personality has no precise meaning and is generally taken to signify a patient's behaviour in its totality. The word, despite its vagueness, is useful for a witness may observe a change in a patient's personality without being able to discern which aspect of the patient's behaviour has deviated from his normal. A history of a change of personality should therefore be accepted although the witness fails to pin-point the change.

Patients are often unaware of changes in their behaviour, intelligence, memory and emotions and, consequently, when a cerebral disease is diagnosed a near-relative should be interviewed for it may emerge that there was evidence of disease prior to the date of onset given by the patient.

CHAPTER XXIII

CEREBRAL SEGMENTAL SIGNS
(Continued)

Seizures

The words 'seizure', 'fit', 'attack' and 'paroxysm' will be taken to be synonymous. Such words refer to the temporal element of properties rather than to the content or quality itself. Thus to speak of a fit of convulsions and a fit of laughing is to use the word 'fit' appropriately although the content of each fit is different. The word 'seizure' or any of its synonyms can be applied to any symptoms or signs provided they last no more than a few hours. It should be noted that to say a patient has a seizure is to say nothing for the word 'seizure' by itself does not signify an appearance. Some other word or words must be used in conjunction with it as, for example, major convulsive seizure.

Seizures are often repeated at regular or irregular intervals and the sign-time graph has therefore a characteristic appearance (Fig. 57). This is a very common graph in clinical medicine and is a most important one. In the majority of cases in clinical neurology an inference of an organic lesion from this graph has a low probability.

The word 'epilepsy' will not be used for three reasons. Epilepsy is defined in a number of ways but a common one is as follows.

> A convulsion is called epilepsy when it is caused by abnormal neuronal discharges in the cerebrum.

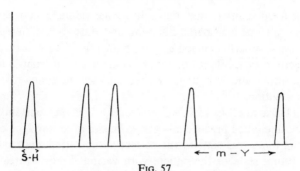

FIG. 57
The Sign-time Graph of a Paroxysmal Disorder.

Let us write this out as a correlative proposition.

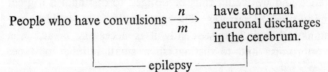

You will see that the definition of epilepsy contains terms which, in routine practice, signify both evidence and inference and objections have previously been raised against this.* The second objection is that the term 'abnormal discharge' does not signify an appearance, observed or imagined, and this alone is enough to condemn the word 'epilepsy' as it is generally used. The third objection is that in the definition the word 'convulsion' is often replaced by a term which signifies another appearance and, as a result, epilepsy is often defined as a seizure which may or may not consist of convulsions. This indicates that convulsions are irrelevant to the definition.

In clinical medicine seizures constitute evidence and the problem really is to decide when two seizures are to be

*A definition cannot, by definition, contain a probability term.

considered similar, and thus given one name, and when they are to be considered different, and thus given different names. You will remember that, with regard to evidence, a decision of similarity or difference depends on what is to be inferred and it is to inferences that we must now turn our attention.

There are four kinds of inferences which we constantly make in clinical practice and these are site of lesion, type of lesion, the future state of the patient without treatment and the future state of the patient with various kinds of treatment. We are, therefore, faced with the problem of dividing seizures into types which will allow four inferences. This is a tall order, for usually one inference requires its own evidence and we would thus be obliged to distinguish a great many types of seizures. The number, in fact, would be unmanageable and consequently it is necessary to accept a compromise and to distinguish a small number of types

THE CLASSIFICATION OF PEOPLE WITH SEIZURES

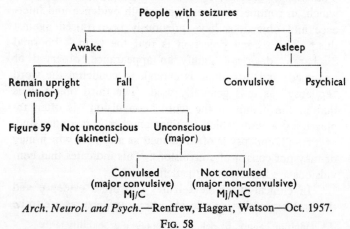

Arch. Neurol. and Psych.—Renfrew, Haggar, Watson—Oct. 1957.

Fig. 58

which, although not the best for each kind of inference we wish to make, is nevertheless fairly satisfactory in routine practice. It is convenient to show the types of seizures in a classification but remember that it is people who are classified and not seizures. Seizures are the properties used in constructing the classification of people. The classification, which is broken into two parts (Figs. 58 and 59), is at first sight a little overwhelming but if we work through it systematically you will find it quite simple.

People with seizures are first divided into those who have their attacks while awake and those who have them while asleep. The first group is divided into two classes on the basis of falling and remaining upright. Being upright means keeping the head and trunk erect and it follows that a patient can sit upright in a chair or in bed. When the patient remains upright the seizure is called minor. Of the people who fall, some are unconscious and some are not. A seizure in which the patient falls unconscious is called major. This group is divided into convulsive and non-convulsive. A convulsion means any muscle action, tonic or clonic, of any muscle whether somatic or visceral and of any degree occurring during the unconscious phase of the seizure. A patient may cry out as he is on the point of falling unconscious and this may be considered as a convulsive movement. Urinary incontinence, however, presents a difficulty. Should the bladder muscles go into spasm the urine is voided and this would be covered by the term ' convulsive '. However, should the muscles of the bladder and sphincter relax, the urine may be voided as a result of gravity. This inhibition of muscular activity occurs in major non-convulsive attacks and it follows that incontinence of urine puts the patient into both the convulsive

63

THE CLASSIFICATION OF PEOPLE WITH SEIZURES

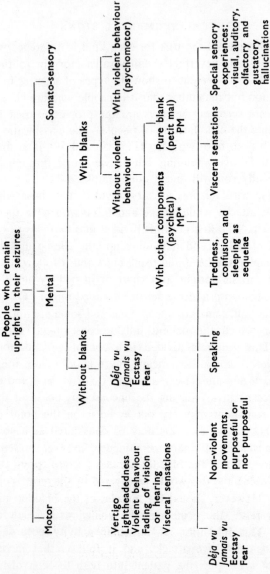

People who remain upright in their seizures

Motor

Vertigo
Lightheadedness
Violent behaviour
Fading of vision or hearing
Visceral sensations

Non-violent movements, purposeful or not purposeful

Déja vu
Jamais vu
Ecstasy
Fear

Mental

Without blanks

Déja vu
Jamais vu
Ecstasy
Fear

Speaking

With blanks

Without violent behaviour

With violent behaviour (psychomotor)

Pure blank (petit mal) PM

With other components (psychical) MP*

Tiredness, confusion and sleeping as sequelae

Visceral sensations

Somato-sensory

Special sensory experiences: visual, auditory, olfactory and gustatory hallucinations

* The abbreviation MP is derived from the initials of the words mental and psychical. It is introduced to draw a distinction between it and the abbreviation PM.

Arch. Neurol. and Psych.—Renfrew, Haggar, Watson.—Oct. 1957.

FIG. 59

and non-convulsive classes. It is, therefore, an irrelevant sign.

A seizure in which the patient falls without losing consciousness is called akinetic. Since it is possible that the patient may lose consciousness and regain it before hitting the ground it may be difficult, if not impossible, to decide whether consciousness has been lost. This, fortunately, is unimportant, for the inferences to be made from akinetic and major non-convulsive seizures are the same. Sometimes a patient may fall because of a myoclonic jerk of the legs and obviously akinetic would not be an appropriate term. Since the falling is incidental to the myoclonus no special name is required.

Seizures occurring during sleep are of two types. One consists of muscle activity while the patient is unconscious and, to distinguish it from major convulsive fits in which falling is essential,* it should be called a sleep convulsive seizure or a sleep convulsion. The other kind of sleep seizure will be mentioned under mental seizures.

There are three types of minor seizures, motor, somato-sensory and mental. The motor attacks, which may be called minor convulsive attacks, consist of involuntary muscle activity of any kind and such terms as ' spasms ', ' twitches ' and ' jerkings ' may be used when they seem appropriate. There is a special kind of activity, already referred to, called myoclonus, in which a limb makes a sharp jerking movement and although this may be repeated several times, many seconds pass between each jerk. In clonic jerking, on the other hand, one jerk immediately follows another. It has been stated that the movements of a

---

* We are in an obvious difficulty with a patient who, while *lying* awake, becomes unconscious and is convulsed. As an exercise you should rearrange the classification so that the term ' major convulsive ' means being unconscious and convulsed. But you will find that you cannot avoid introducing another class.

minor convulsive seizure are involuntary and to this it may be added that they are also purposeless. Similar remarks would seem relevant to the movements of a major convulsive seizure but they are superfluous in view of the fact that the patient is unconscious (grade 1).*

Somato-sensory seizures consist of spontaneous feelings in any part of the body. It is advisable to divide this group into two classes, one in which the patient feels that a limb is moving (although it is in fact stationary) or that it is growing in size, and the other in which the patient experiences tingling feelings or pins and needles. The reason for this division will be seen later.

Of the minor seizures the mental type is the most common. Mental seizures are first divided into two types on the basis of the presence or absence of a mental blank. This mental blank, or blank for short, is very important and we must try to make the definition as precise as possible.

A mental blank† is a state of unresponsiveness and amnesia. Unresponsiveness means that the patient does not respond, at least not rationally, to questions and commands. Amnesia means, in the context of the definition, a lack of memory for events occurring outside the patient during the seizure. The patient may not remember his mental experiences either but this is irrelevant to the definition. An amnesia for mental experiences during the seizure is, however, important clinically, for this is invariably associated with an amnesia for external events, so that if the former is the only evidence available the latter may be inferred from

---

* A patient who does not respond to pain and yet makes purposeful, and possibly violent, movements is in unconscious grade 4 according to our definition of this term.

† This is a curious mental state. To distinguish it from unconsciousness, to which it has obvious similarities, it might be advisable to make the property *unable to maintain the upright posture* part of the definition of unconscious grades 1, 2 and 3.

it. It should be noted that a witness is required for the identification of unresponsiveness while the patient himself may be able to describe the amnesia.

It must be emphasised that a blank means *both* unresponsiveness and amnesia. A patient who is sulking may be said to be unresponsive and a patient with a hysterical fugue has an amnesia. The former has no amnesia and the latter is responsive during the fugue. The terms ' unresponsiveness ' and ' amnesia ' must be used with care. Should you shut your eyes you can hardly be accused later of not remembering what you would have seen if your eyes had been opened. Similarly, should you cover your ears you can hardly be expected to remember what someone said to you, nor can you be described as being unresponsive to his questions and commands. Some patients describe attacks in which their vision fades or in which they voluntarily close their eyes. Other patients say that in their attacks peoples' voices fade away in the distance and they cannot hear clearly what they are saying. In all such cases close questioning will reveal that the patients have some memory of external events during their attacks and consequently the terms ' amnesia ' and ' mental blank ' cannot be strictly applied.

Mental seizures without blanks may consist of strange mental experiences. The patient may have a curious feeling of familiarity in surroundings which are unfamiliar or he may have a feeling of unfamiliarity in familiar surroundings. Sometimes a variation of these experiences, which may be called *deja vu,* consists of a feeling that new events which are being witnessed in the present have been previously observed. Rarely a patient may feel that events are moving with great rapidity or very slowly. Another type of mental experience consists of feelings of extreme pleasure (ecstasy) or displeasure, the latter amounting to horror or fear. With regard to the latter it must be realised that attacks of any sort, provided the patient remains conscious, provoke, as a rule, a not unnatural fear. The fear during a mental seizure is easily identified if it forms the entire content of the attack, for in this case it has no apparent provocation. It may also be identified by the patient who may say that it has a strange quality quite unlike that of any feeling of horror or terror which he has experienced in what, for the moment, may be described as normal circumstances. Quite often, unfortunately, the patient is unable to describe his mental experiences, not because he is inarticulate but because the experiences are indescribable in the sense that the language does not contain appropriate words. The words we have at our disposal, of course, signify only common experiences.

Mental seizures with blanks are of three types and these will now be enumerated.

1. *Psychomotor seizures.**—In these attacks the patient behaves in a destructive way towards people and property and during the attacks he is not, as it were, amenable to reason; afterwards he has no recollection of his behaviour. The last part of this definition constitutes the mental blank. This kind of attack has obvious medico-legal implications.

2. *Petit mal.*—This kind of seizure consists of unresponsiveness and a total amnesia, that is, the patient remembers nothing of external events or of his experiences during the attacks. He exhibits no movements except perhaps a fluttering of the eyelids, fumbling with the hands or myoclonic jerks. As an aid to memory you should think of petit mal as nothing but a pure blank.

* The various definitions given are somewhat different to those given in standard textbooks.

3. *Psychical seizures.*—This kind of seizure consists of a mental blank (remember that according to the definition the amnesia must be at least partial but may be total) and in addition there is one or more of a great variety of features which are enumerated in the classification. The names given to these features are, for the most part, self-explanatory, but the non-violent actions deserve some amplification. During a psychical seizure the patient may walk about in a fairly normal fashion or he may perform strange and sometimes embarrassing acts. He may, for example, stamp a foot or turn around in one spot. He may undress or embrace whoever happens to be near. Common actions are those of chewing or swallowing. Speaking is a very common feature and some effort may have to be made to elicit this evidence since the patient and his relatives may try to suppress it on the ground that it suggests insanity. Speaking may take one of several forms. The patient may speak jargon, mumble incoherently, sing a song, or make a statement which, although a proposition, is either absurd or is completely out of context with a conversation he may have been having. Almost invariably the patient has no recollection of having spoken, although an occasional patient may remember a desire to speak and may even recall that his statement would have been nonsense.

Psychical seizures may occur during sleep. The patient may sit up or get up and thereafter behave in the way described above. It is evident that the seizure may be confused with sleep-walking but the distinction is easily made, for a patient can be roused from sleep-walking but not from a psychical seizure.

It is important to draw a clear distinction between petit mal and psychical seizures, for the treatment of the two conditions and the inferences to be drawn are very different. The definitions will not be altered but some relevant remarks can, nevertheless, be made and these will be enumerated. You should use this list as an exercise in identifying correlative and definitive propositions.

1. Petit mal rarely continues after the age of 25 years and even more rarely begins after this age. Psychical seizures begin at any age and continue to any age.

2. A patient may be aware of being in a psychical seizure but he cannot be aware of being in a petit mal. This is equivalent to saying that the amnesia in a psychical seizure may be partial but must be total in a petit mal. A patient with petit mal may be aware of having had an attack because he has missed part of a conversation or he has forgotten what he was doing but he cannot remember being in the attack. It must be admitted that some patients with petit mal know that they have had an attack but cannot explain how they come to know this.

3. A petit mal rarely lasts more than 30 seconds while a psychical seizure may last several hours.

4. A patient may feel a psychical seizure coming on but he cannot feel a petit mal coming on. The remarks given under 2 are relevant here.

5. A patient may have symptoms such as sleepiness after a psychical seizure but not after a petit mal.

6. Patients with petit mal who are not being treated nearly always have several attacks a day. Patients with psychical seizures who are untreated may have several attacks a day or only one in a life-time.

7. Patients with psychical seizures often complain of a poor memory apart from the attacks. This is not so with petit mal.

Occasionally the distinction between petit mal and psychical seizures may be difficult since the necessary evidence is not forthcoming. Sometimes, too, the patient may be subject to both kinds of attacks so that the history-taking may be difficult. Quite often the mental experiences of a psychical seizure may be so brief, perhaps a split second, that a mental blank cannot be identified with confidence. Although it may be difficult to distinguish between a mental seizure without a blank and a psychical seizure, there is no difficulty in distinguishing both from a petit mal.

With regard to the classification of patients with seizures, three points must be noted. First, it may be difficult to classify the patient for want of evidence. Second, a patient cannot have two types of seizures simultaneously, that is to say, at any one moment he can only be put into one class. And third, a patient may have two or more types of seizures at different times, either in rapid sequence or at widely spaced intervals. Always remember that in all scientific classifications an object is not put into a class for the purpose of applying a name. It is put into a class for the purpose of making inferences and if an object can be put into two or more classes of the same classification at different times so much the better, for more inferences can be made. Returning to seizures, it is not uncommon for a patient to have a rapid succession of seizures. For example, he may begin with a psychical seizure, proceed immediately to a major convulsive attack and then end with a psycho-motor fit. Or he may start with a minor convulsive fit and pass to a major convulsive attack. All sorts of combinations occur. It should perhaps be added that at different times a patient may have psychical seizures and mental seizures without blanks.

The aura and sequel of seizures

It is customary to divide seizures into three parts whenever this can be conveniently done. The middle part is usually the period during which consciousness is lost or impaired or during which convulsions occur. Quite often the first and third parts, called respectively the aura and sequel, can be described as seizures according to the classification, but for the moment we will consider symptoms of another sort. The aura, for example, may consist of vertigo, of lightheaded feelings or of feelings in the abdomen and chest. Indeed, a common aura is a feeling beginning in the abdomen and then radiating into the chest and head. There is a great variety of such symptoms and although they are not important diagnostically, since they cannot be used as cerebral segmental signs, they are of value to the patient provided they give him enough time to get into a position of safety.

The sequelae may be more distressing and disabling than the convulsion or psychical seizure which precedes them. The patient may feel ill for a few hours or days. He may feel sleepy and may fall into a deep sleep for several hours and, although he may be roused, he may fall asleep again. Apart from sleepiness and drowsiness the patient may exhibit mild mental confusion for a period lasting usually for minutes or hours but occasionally, in the case of major convulsive seizures, for a few days. Headache and vomiting are common sequels and after a convulsion the patient often complains of muscular aches and pains. An important sequel is weakness of the limbs on one side following a convulsion, for if this weakness persists for more than 48 hours an organic cerebral lesion is highly probable.

After a major non-convulsive attack the patient may shiver as a result of cold or fear and if care is not taken it may be supposed that the patient has had a major convulsive attack. On close questioning it will be discovered that the shivering associated with a major non-convulsive attack occurs during the recovery phase and not during the period of unconsciousness.

The duration of seizures

While major and minor convulsive seizures, somato-sensory and psychomotor seizures must last at least a few seconds, since otherwise they could scarcely be identified, petit mal and psychical seizures may last only a fraction of a second. On the other hand, all seizures, with the exception of petit mal and akinetic seizures, may last several hours.

The frequency of seizures

There are four ways of reckoning the frequency of seizures.

1. The minimum number of attacks occurring in a specified period (a day, week, month or year).

2. The maximum number of attacks occurring in a specified period.

3. The average number of attacks occurring in a specified period.

4. The longest period during which the patient remains free of attacks.

The last method is the best although this and method 3 can be conveniently combined. For example, a patient who has an average of four attacks a month and can miss a week but not a month can be said to have four attacks a month.

The following code is a helpful method of abbreviation.

1 + /D   The patient has at least one attack every day calculated on the basis of the previous two weeks. One attack may follow immediately on another.

1 + /W   The patient has at least one attack every week calculated on the basis of the previous month.

1 + /M   The patient has at least one attack every month calculated on the basis of the previous six months.

1 + /Y   The patient has at least one attack every year calculated on the basis of the previous few years.

A patient who has had 12 attacks in one day but only on one day in a year would be coded as 12/Y. The code indicates that the patient enjoys months of freedom but not how the attacks are spaced. The latter point, although important in the patient's everyday life, is irrelevant in therapeutic management. A period of freedom from attacks lasting at least a year may be called a remission.

Seizures as cerebral segmental signs

There is a bewildering variety of seizures and all are caused by the cerebrum, for in the absence of the cerebrum no movements occur and no feelings are experienced, not even headache, backache or indigestion. This causal correlation is, of course, worthless and we are obliged, for practical purposes, to divide seizures into two broad types. From the first we can infer organic cerebral lesions with a probability which, although low, is not negligible and this low probability we will refer to as a working probability. From the second, inferences of organic cerebral lesions are so low that they can be safely ignored. Examples will make this clear. From a major convulsive fit we would infer an organic cerebral lesion with a low probability but, nevertheless, we would pursue an investigation in an effort to produce evidence which would raise or lower this probability. On the other hand, from a transient pain in the stomach we would infer an organic cerebral lesion with such a low probability that further investigation of a cerebral lesion would be futile. The numerical level at which a non-working probability changes to a working one depends on the importance of the inference and on the attitude of the clinician.

Seizures which allow working probability inferences of organic cerebral lesions may be called cerebral segmental signs. Some of the seizures in the classification are of this nature and some are not, as will later be seen.

Causes of seizures

A seizure of a particular type, being a sign, is a reflection of the site of a lesion rather than of its type. As one might expect, any kind of lesion, whether histological or chemical, provided it is in an appropriate site, can cause a particular type of seizure.

It is also to be expected that seizures as an effect must have a chain of causal properties which correlate with them. Some links in the chain may be situated in the cerebrum but others may be outside it. Thus, circumstances which provoke fear or pain may cause attacks. Similarly, circumstances associated with loss of sleep, over-work, excitement and anxiety may act as causal properties.

Inferences from seizures

It cannot be too strongly emphasised that seizures must be considered as evidence and only as evidence. Evidence can never be an end in itself and it is on the inferences that we must centre our attention. As has previously been indicated inferences should be placed under four headings. The remarks to be made about convulsions and psychical seizures occurring while the patient is awake are also applicable to those attacks occurring during sleep.

1. The site of lesion: Major and minor convulsive attacks beginning in, or restricted to, one side indicate a

lesion in the opposite cerebral hemisphere in the region of the motor cortex. Similarly, a somato-sensory seizure which is restricted to one side indicates a lesion in the opposite sensory cortex. A psychical seizure allows an inference of a temporal lobe lesion (and for this reason it is often called a temporal lobe seizure) but it is not possible to infer the side. It might have been thought that speaking would suggest the dominant hemisphere but this proves not to be the case. Generalised convulsions, petit mal, akinetic, major non-convulsive and psychomotor seizures do not allow inferences of site.

2. The type of lesion: Major and minor convulsive, somato-sensory and psychical seizures allow working probability inferences of histological lesions in the cerebrum. With regard to somato-sensory attacks, inferences from tingling feelings have a negligible probability, while inferences from space feelings have a working probability. The probability of histological lesions with all the attacks mentioned is about 1 in 100 in young adults and rises progressively in middle and old age.

Major non-convulsive, akinetic and psychomotor seizures, mental seizures without blanks and petit mal do not allow working probability inferences of cerebral histological lesions.

Major convulsive, major non-convulsive seizures and psychomotor seizures allow very low probability inferences of chemical cerebral lesions, anoxia and hypoglycaemia being the commonest. Whether the probability is to be considered a working one is a matter of doubt. For example, does a major non-convulsive attack (sometimes called fainting or syncope) justify a search for remote causes of cerebral anoxia? Some clinicians would perhaps reply that if fainting is caused by pain, fear, cold or prolonged standing it is unnecessary to search further for a cause but in the absence of these provocations an investigation of the blood and cardiovascular system should be undertaken. The problem is a difficult one and you will hear many points of view.

3. The future state of the patient without treatment: It can be taken as a general rule that with all types of seizures the more frequent they have been in the past and the longer the period during which they have occurred the more likely are they to occur in the future. Puberty, the menopause, pregnancy and the weeks after a confinement are periods when the attacks may be more frequent. At least half the female patients who have seizures about once a month have their attacks in relation to the menstrual periods. Some patients may have their attacks less frequently during a pregnancy.

Petit mal seizures nearly always disappear before the age of 25 years although, unfortunately, they may be replaced by major convulsive attacks.

Apart from the future frequency of seizures many inferences can be made which are relevant to the patient's everyday life. Patients who are subject to a periodic loss or impairment of consciousness may be killed or injured if they drive vehicles, tend dangerous machinery, go up ladders or otherwise put themselves in a position of danger. Frequent seizures of any type may impair the working efficiency of a patient and the appearance of his seizures may be distressing to those who happen to witness them. Psychical seizures, as has already been mentioned, may be a source of great embarrassment and bring the patient into contact with the police. The latter event will almost certainly occur when the patient is subject to psychomotor seizures unless he is previously brought under medical care. It is clear that the inferences which are to be made are a matter of common sense and depend on the type and frequency of the seizures, the presence or absence of an aura which gives the patient an opportunity of avoiding danger and the particular environment in which the patient spends his life.

4. The future state of the patient with treatment: Major and minor convulsive, somato-sensory and psychical seizures often become less frequent when appropriate treatment is instituted. Petit mal also shows a good response although it should be noted that it requires a different kind of treatment from the seizures which were first mentioned.

Akinetic, major non-convulsive and psychomotor seizures have a poor response to drug therapy. The response of mental seizures without blanks (*déja vu, etc.*) has not been investigated. It is probably poor although treatment should always be given a trial.

Other seizures

There are three types of attacks which deserve a few remarks.

Narcolepsy.—This kind of attack consists of sleep preceded by an intense and often irresistible desire to sleep. The sleep may last several hours and may occur several times a day. In this connection sleep is an appropriate word for the patient can be roused.

Cataplexy.—This attack consists of inhibition of the somatic musculature with the result that the patient may fall to the ground. The muscular weakness is caused by emotion often pleasant and rarely unpleasant but does not occur unless the patient gives expression to the emotion. Narcolepsy and cataplexy often occur together, although of course at different times, and are thought to be related to lesions in the hypothalamic region.

Hysterical seizures.—Clinicians often say that certain seizures are hysterical although whether the word ' hysterical ' signifies the appearance of the seizures or their cause or both is never made clear. You are well advised never to use the word hysteria until you have been qualified for several years and until you have become an expert diagnostician. You will remain on safe ground if you restrict yourself, with regard to a certain kind of seizure, to the statement that the inference of an organic cerebral lesion is extremely low. You may add in some cases that with psychotherapy the patient will probably improve but beyond this you should not venture.

The kind of attack which will tempt you to use the word ' hysteria ' is one in which the patient is unresponsive and behaves violently but not destructively and in which the movements are purposeful. This kind of seizure is rare and you should take care to distinguish it from major convulsive and psychomotor seizures.

Conclusion

This account of seizures may seem to be unduly elaborate. The subject, however, is a difficult one as you will no doubt soon discover for yourself. Moreover, in no branch of clinical medicine have clinicians become the slaves of words more than in that relating to seizures.

It may occur to you that the avoidance of the word ' epilepsy ' may give rise to embarrassing situations with patients and colleagues alike. You will find, however, that patients will not be upset if you remark that you do not use the word ' epilepsy ' on the ground that it has no scientific meaning. You will also find that they will be grateful if you add that the problem, it seems to you, is not to give seizures a name, for any name would do, but to find their cause if possible, to predict the future and to prescribe treatment.

Skill in the diagnosis of seizures obviously rests on history-taking both from patients and witnesses. You should insist on descriptions which are completely free from such terms as blackouts, faints and dizziness for the meaning of such terms is vague. Lay witnesses often speak in terms of inferences rather than of evidence and if the clinician is not on his guard he may be completely led astray. For example, a witness will often say that a patient's limbs were rigid or stiff when he means only that they were straight. In taking histories, work through the classification point by point, asking direct questions rather than allowing irrelevancies to obscure the issue. Remember that the aim of history-taking is not to get a *complete* description but only to get sufficient evidence to put the patient into one of the classes of the classification you happen to be using at the time.

The names of seizures used above are those generally accepted. The following synonyms should be noted.

> Major convulsive and grand mal
> Psychical seizure and temporal lobe seizure
> Minor motor, focal motor and Jacksonian seizure.

The definitions given are a little more precise than those usually used. The inclusion of the mental blank in the definition of psychical seizure is unorthodox but to omit it means that any periodic odd mental state or behaviour has to be called a psychical seizure. The class would therefore become too large to be useful in medical practice.

If you insist on retaining the term epilepsy you should only use it when you have identified the following kinds of seizures.

Major convulsive, minor motor, psychical, psycho-motor, petit mal, sleep convulsion and sleep psychical.

The use of the term epilepsy with regard to other types of seizures is controversial. You will note that the term epilepsy covers several types of seizures and consequently it does not convey precise information. If to correct this the type of seizure is added to the term epilepsy you will see that the term epilepsy does not give added information. In short, epilepsy is not a useful word even if it obeyed the rules of definition.

CHAPTER XXIV

HEADACHE, FACIAL PAIN AND VERTIGO

Headache

Headache is a word used by lay people and to them it means any disagreeable feeling, painful or otherwise, in the region of the vault of the skull.

Causes of headache: Since it is impossible to provoke pain by experimental stimulation of the central nervous system it is assumed that pathological processes only cause headache when they involve, directly or indirectly, other tissues of the head. Infective and neoplastic lesions may irritate tissues immediately adjacent, while a lesion which increases the pressure of intracranial contents, a so-called space-occupying lesion, may produce pain by the compression or traction of tissues nearby or at a distance. Only a small proportion of headaches, however, are caused by such lesions.

There is evidence that pain may be provoked by dilatation of cranial arteries including the circle of Willis and the proximal but not the distal parts of the cerebral arteries. Possibly the headache associated with toxic conditions may be explained in this way and possibly, too, many headaches for which no organic cause can be found. The dilatation which we are considering at the moment is within normal limits and since there are no histological changes it cannot be called an organic lesion.

Some clinicians claim that there are many other causes of headache among which are refractive errors, sinusitis,*

---

* Chronic sinusitis has probably been overrated as a cause of headache and facial pain.

carious teeth, unerupted teeth and cervical spondylosis. Let us consider the first as an example of the group. When headache disappears with the wearing of spectacles you are apt to claim that poor vision is the cause of headache. However, to establish poor vision as a cause of headache, it would be necessary to observe two groups of patients both of which were treated in exactly the same way except that in one group vision was corrected whereas in the other it was not. As a result of this experiment two propositions could be formulated as follows.

$$\text{People} \begin{cases} \text{with headache and poor vision and who wear spectacles which do not correct vision} & \xrightarrow{\frac{n}{m}} \text{continue to have headache.} \\ \\ \text{with headache and who wear spectacles which correct vision} & \xrightarrow{\frac{n-q}{m}} \text{continue to have headache.} \end{cases}$$

If there is a significant difference in the probabilities of the two propositions then poor vision is a cause of headache. As an exercise you should write a pair of propositions with the inference *stop having headache* which would show that wearing spectacles is a cure for headache.

Clinicians who maintain that poor vision is a cause of headache do not take the trouble to plan an experiment with a control group but simply assume that their conviction, based on the observation that some headaches disappear when spectacles are worn, is proof that they are right.

Head injury, no matter its severity, is often followed by headache which may persist for long periods. In only a small number is the headache due to an organic lesion produced by trauma. Anxiety and worry, which are often

83

considered to be a cause of headache, will be discussed in a later chapter.

The routine investigation of headache: Headache caused by toxaemia does not present a difficult diagnostic problem for the headache is usually only one of several symptoms produced by the toxaemia. To simplify the following discussion we will omit headaches caused by toxaemia so that we are left with headache due to space-occupying lesions and headache for which no organic cause can be found. Intracranial infections will, for convenience, be included in the first group. In the second group we will include those headaches which some clinicians believe are due to refractive errors, carious teeth and so on, on the ground that such abnormalities have not been proved, to our satisfaction, to have a causal relation with headache.

Intracranial space-occupying lesions are not common in the general population so that the inference of such lesions from headache have a low probability. The presence of neurological and radiological signs, of course, increase the probability greatly and for this reason any patient complaining of headache deserves a thorough clinical examination. Unfortunately, or rather fortunately, most examinations prove negative and the clinician is often left wondering when he should institute special neuro-radiological investigations and when he should persuade a patient to submit himself to repeated clinical examinations over a long period of time. The history given by the patient offers some guide and in Figure 60 are listed properties, in order of importance, which raise or lower the probability of a space-occupying lesion.

The aim, of course, is to end with a probability of a space-occupying lesion which could be described as a working level or a negligible level. This unfortunately

THE INFERENCE OF AN ORGANIC LESION FROM HEADACHE

PROPERTIES WHICH LOWER THE PROBABILITY OF A SPACE-OCCUPYING LESION

	SCORE
Headache which consists of a disagreeable feeling as opposed to pain Examples are a pressing, creeping and crushing feeling	−2
Headaches which are of long duration (over 2 years)...	−1
Headaches which have a throbbing, shooting or stabbing quality	−1
Headaches which are paroxysmal with long periods of freedom	−1
Headaches which are localised to a small area of the head	−1

PROPERTIES WHICH RAISE THE PROBABILITY OF A SPACE OCCUPYING LESION

Headaches which are provoked by coughing as distinct from being aggravated by coughing	+3
Headaches which are painful and have an aching quality ...	+2
Headaches which are of short duration (less than 2 years)	+1
Headaches which are continuous or paroxysmal with short periods of freedom (hours or days)	+1

Fig. 60

presents a very difficult problem. To take the edge off it a scoring system is shown in Figure 60. A positive score is considered to give a working level while a zero or negative score is considered to give a negligible level. However, the definition of a working level will vary with circumstances. The level will be fairly low for a general practitioner who is debating whether to send a patient to a specialist but fairly high for a specialist who is debating whether to submit a patient to arteriography or ventriculography. It may be added at this point that the probability of an organic lesion is considerably raised if the patient looks ill between headaches. More will be said of this in connection with neoplasms.

Migraine.—Most headaches have no organic cause. From this large group clinicians have singled out one type and given it the name ' migraine '. Migraine is a name for evidence but unfortunately there is no general agreement about the definition. It is often said to be headache which begins in or is confined to one side of the head and is associated with visual disturbances. It is also said to be associated with vomiting and to run in families. Clinicians, however, pay only lip-service to this definition for they apply the term when one or two of the above elements are absent.

The visual disturbances show a good deal of variation. They may consist of a partial or complete loss of vision in one part of the visual field, often a homonymous hemianopic defect and rarely a total peripheral loss (tubular vision). Sometimes the patient sees coloured spots and lines which often assume a zig-zag appearance. Some patients admit only a blurring of vision while others give a picturesque description of the visual disturbance saying, perhaps, that it is like looking through glass with water running down it. Indeed there is an infinite variety of visual experiences. In one patient, too, there may be some variation and the visual disturbances may alternate between the two sides. These visual experiences last only a matter of minutes, rarely more than an hour, and as a rule, but not invariably, precede the headache.

Occasionally the visual disturbances are associated with or are replaced by paraesthesiae which occur mostly in the hand and face of one side although in one patient they may alternate between the two sides. The patient will often claim that the hand becomes weak but usually he means that the hand has become clumsy or useless. On close questioning it will be discovered that the clumsiness is due to a loss of space sense. If weakness can be verified an organic lesion should be seriously considered. The paraesthesiae, like the visual disturbances, last only a few minutes and occur prior to the headache in most instances.

A few patients with headache complain of difficulty in speaking at the beginning of an attack and this as a rule is associated with paraesthesiae. A feeling of sickness or vomiting is a fairly common accompaniment of headache and may occur at any stage of the attack. It will be seen later in the chapter on neoplasms that vomiting raises the probability of increased intracranial pressure so that in any patient it should not be too lightly dismissed. Nevertheless, if headache with vomiting has occurred over many years with long periods of freedom, the probability of an organic lesion is negligible.

Of the many patients with headaches not due to an organic lesion, a few have all the elements given in the above description of migraine. Some have one or two of the elements and some have none. This would seem to introduce a diagnostic problem but this problem disappears if you remember that the name attached to a headache is quite unimportant. It is the inferences which are important and these inferences are the same whether you think the term ' migraine ' can justifiably be applied or not. Indeed if the problem troubles you, you should stop using the term ' migraine ' altogether and speak only of headaches.

Taking a history from a patient with headache.— Questions should be put to the patient which will reveal the various features already mentioned. Most of the questions will be answered accurately but there is one question which is frequently answered carelessly and this is the one referring to duration. Most patients date their headache from the time at which it began to worry or disable them, from the time at which they reported to their doctor or from the time at which analgesics failed to give relief. Unfortunately the lay public divide headaches into two types, one which they suppose is of serious import and the other which they call normal headaches. In the great majority of cases, patients who have headaches not due to organic lesions will admit that they have had normal headaches prior to their present headache. In questioning a patient about duration do not ask if he previously suffered from, was bothered by or was subject to headache for you must appreciate that none of these terms apply, in the lay mind, to normal headache. To repeat, adults who complain at first of recent headache will nearly always admit headaches for many years. The problem, of course, is to decide whether the recent headache is a continuation or exacerbation of a long-standing headache but, fortunaately, in only a small number of cases is the problem a difficult one.

Similarly, adults who give a history of recent continuous headache will frequently admit previous paroxysmal headache, and adults who complain of migrainous headache will admit previous headache to which the term ' migraine ' could not justifiably be applied.

Conclusion.—Only the inference of an organic lesion has so far received attention. Clearly we ought to be thinking in terms of prognosis with and without treatment. As in the case of seizures previously described, it can be taken as a rule that the longer the duration and the more frequent the headache the more likely is the patient to continue to have headache in the future. The prognosis with treatment is, however, much more difficult. The truth is that some patients get relief with various kinds of therapy which can act only as placebos while other patients get no relief even with powerful analgesics. It has to be concluded that there is no way of classifying patients with a view to making inferences of response to treatment.

Facial pain*

Pains in the face, eye and mouth are generally focal and are caused by nearby inflammatory and neoplastic lesions which may be obvious or may require careful investigation if they are to be demonstrated. Pains which may be considered to be neurological are rarely caused by an organic neurological lesion. Only two distinct types are worth describing.

Tic douloureux.—This is a name for evidence. It should not be considered to be synonymous with trigeminal neuralgia since the latter term covers all kinds of facial pain.

Tic douloureux is a condition which is not caused by an organic lesion and occurs only in elderly people. It is confined to one side of the face and is most common in the 2nd and 3rd divisions of the 5th nerve. It is never confined to the 1st division although this division may rarely be affected in association with the other divisions. The pain is distinctly paroxysmal and lasts only a few seconds. The paroxysms may be repeated at intervals of only a few seconds for a matter of minutes or hours but in most cases they are separated by minutes, hours or days. There may be repeated paroxysms over weeks or

* Pain in the face and elsewhere is sometimes a sequel of herpes zoster. This condition will be included in your course in dermatology.

months with intervals of complete freedom lasting weeks or months. As the condition progresses, however, the periods of freedom become shorter.

A paroxysm of pain may begin in the 2nd or 3rd division. It may start at one spot in the face or mouth and then shoot over a short distance within the division or into a neighbouring division. The pain is intense (it is too brief to have an aching or throbbing quality) and it may be so distressing that the patient remains rigid and motionless with the face twisted and the hands held up to, but not touching, the face.

Frequently the pain is triggered by touching certain areas of the face and mouth, the so-called trigger areas, and the patient is careful to avoid contacting these areas as far as possible. Washing, shaving, a draught of air, eating and talking may provoke pain and consequently the patient's life is far from a happy one.

Two important points have to be remembered. There are no neurological signs and the pain never spreads beyond the territory of the 5th nerve.

Middle-aged adults may get pain similar to that described above in association with disseminated sclerosis. When the pain begins during the course of this disease there is no diagnostic difficulty but when the pain precedes it, as it occasionally does, the clinician may be at a loss for a diagnosis. For this reason, with patients under the age of 50 years, the possibility of disseminated sclerosis should always be kept in mind.

Migrainous neuralgia.—This condition occurs in adults of any age. The pain has a throbbing, gnawing or burning quality and is continuous, sometimes for years. It may be localised to quite a small area of the face or be widespread over the head, face, mouth and neck on one or both sides.

The pain is roughly in the distribution of cranial arteries which may be found to be tender on pressure.

The term 'migrainous neuralgia', which is a name for evidence, has the advantage that it reminds us that the facial pain is no more than a headache in the face.* Indeed most patients with this condition give a long history of headache prior to the facial pain.

You should take care to distinguish migrainous neuralgia from tic douloureux and temporal arteritis, diagnostic problems which are quite easy.

Paroxysmal pain may occur in the globe of the eye or behind it. This pain may be associated with headache or facial pain and, if it is considered to have neurological significance, presents a similar problem with regard to the inference of an organic lesion. Again a long history with long periods of freedom and the absence of neurological signs reduce the probability of an organic lesion to a negligible level.

Vertigo

Vertigo means an illusion of movement. It may consist of a feeling that the subject is moving or that his environment is moving. The kind of movement is irrelevant to the definition. Usually, however, it is rotatory, the rotation being in the horizontal plane with the patient standing. Less commonly it is in the vertical plane. Many other kinds of movement are possible, such as a to-and-fro movement in either plane and a feeling that the ground is rising or that the patient is falling. Occasionally the patient feels that he is walking to one side.

Vertigo is nearly always paroxysmal and lasts only minutes. Rarely it lasts for hours and days.

* Why the term headache should apply only to pain above the eyebrows is something of a mystery.

In describing vertigo patients generally use the words 'dizzy' and 'dizziness'. Unfortunately dizziness is not synonymous with vertigo for the former includes, in the mind of a patient, ataxia and a light-headed feeling. In taking a history the patient has to be asked specifically if he has a feeling of movement. It is advisable to ask him to describe the movement, not that the kind of movement has any neurological significance but his ability to give a description is verification that he has an illusion of movement.

Vertigo, unless it is extremely mild, is associated with incoordination of movement and this is especially noticeable on walking. Usually the patient has to sit or lie down until the vertigo subsides. If the vertigo is severe and sudden the patient may be precipitated to the ground. Movements of the head may aggravate the vertigo and when the vertigo has subsided the movements may continue to provoke it. A feeling of sickness and vomiting are common accompaniments and nystagmus, in addition to the ataxia, is present on examination. Occasionally headache precedes, accompanies or follows the vertigo and rarely a patient may have a major non-convulsive or convulsive seizure after the attack.

Rotational vertigo is a segmental sign to the labyrinth, vestibular nerve and nucleus and the cause of the vertigo may lie at any point on this segment. It is generally held that, in most cases, the lesion is in the labyrinth but this is a matter of speculation since pathological studies have been performed in only a few cases. It is probable that rapid structural or chemical changes in the vestibular nerve or nucleus are required for the production of vertigo when the lesions are so situated. Thus sudden vascular insufficiency of the brain-stem, a rapidly developing brain-stem encephalitis or demyelinating disease may provoke vertigo. More peripherally, sudden alterations in the endolymph system of the labyrinths are probably required. Neoplasms do not cause vertigo although rarely a patient with a tumour will complain of vertigo. Certainly vertigo as an isolated sign does not justify a neurosurgical investigation.

Nerve deafness and tinnitus are often associated with paroxysmal vertigo. They may precede or follow the vertigo by an interval of years. When all three symptoms are present the term 'Ménière's syndrome' can be applied. This obviously is a name for evidence and does not imply a cause. Nevertheless it is usually assumed that structural changes in the vestibular and auditory parts of the inner ear are responsible. Deafness, however, may be caused by a tumour of the 8th nerve and this possibility must be kept in mind when a nerve deafness has been established. A useful distinction between an 8th nerve tumour and changes in the labyrinth is that ataxia is only present with the latter when the patient is vertiginous while, with the former, the patient may be ataxic (cerebellar) although he has no trace of vertigo. It perhaps follows that, with an 8th nerve tumour, the patient is persistently ataxic while, with a labyrinthine disorder, the ataxia is intermittent. It is therefore advisable in every patient who presents with ataxia to determine whether the ataxia occurs independently of vertigo or only in association with it.

Non-rotational vertigo, that is, a feeling of falling, of the ground rising or of a feeling of movement towards one side, has doubtful clinical significance. It is not associated with organic disease and the site of the functional disorder is a matter of pure speculation.

CHAPTER XXV

VISION AND EYE MOVEMENTS

Visual field defects

To bring the visual pathways into line with the motor and somatic sensory pathways we will consider the segmental tracts to include the optic nerves and chiasma while the optic tracts and radiations we will consider to be the long tracts.

As with other sensory pathways the inference of site of lesion follows from the distribution of the visual loss. Before describing these visual defects, however, it is necessary to say something about testing vision.

Central vision (or macular or foveal vision) is tested by asking the patient to read print (Snellen type or Jaeger type). This examination is only important in neurology when it directs your attention to a defect of central vision. The best test of peripheral vision is performed on a Bjerrum screen. This is a black screen which is illuminated by a source of light behind and above the patient who sits at a distance of two metres from the screen with his eyes at the same level as the centre of the screen. A small white target is fixed in the centre of the screen as an aid to the patient in directing his gaze towards the centre. One eye is covered while the other is tested. A white target, the smallest being 2 mm., is fixed to the end of a black handle and the examiner then moves it from the periphery of the screen towards the centre until the patient states that he is aware of it with his peripheral vision. The test is repeated in different parts of the screen. It is convenient

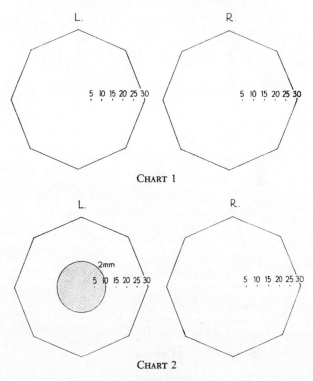

CHART 1

CHART 2

FIG. 61
Charts of Visual Fields.
Chart 1. Normal Fields. Chart 2. A Central Scotoma.

to have the screen marked with black threads which indicate the angle subtended by each point and the centre at
the eye. Thus there are threads at intervals of 5° up to 30°.
The results of the test are transferred to a chart which is
similarly graded and the points joined by a line called an
isopter. The angle at which a 2 mm. target is seen varies
with the illumination of the screen but is usually about 25°.

95

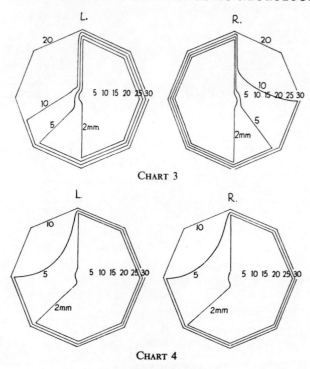

CHART 3

CHART 4

FIG. 61 (*contd.*)
Charts of Visual Fields.
Chart 3. A Bitemporal Hemianopia. Chart 4. A Homo-
nymous Hemianopia.

If, in part of the visual field, the patient cannot see the
2 mm. target until, say, the 15° point is reached the
examiner must use larger targets in an effort to discover
the smallest target which can be seen in the defective area.
The test really has two aims. The first is to demonstrate
a defect in the visual field and the second is to demonstrate
the degree of defect. It is the distribution or shape of the

96

defect, however, rather than its severity which allows an inference of site of lesion.

Ophthalmologists also use a perimeter for testing visual fields but this has no advantage in neurology and has the disadvantage that a slight defect may be overlooked. It is useful in neurology to test the visual fields by a method called the method of confrontation. Here the patient sits at a distance of about two feet from the examiner. Both close one eye while each fixes his gaze on the open eye of the other. The test object is a white-headed hatpin about 2-3 mm. in diameter and this is fixed to a wooden stick or the handle of a tendon hammer. The examiner slowly brings the pin in from the periphery in a plane mid-way between himself and the patient until the patient states that he is aware of it with his peripheral vision. It is preferable that the patient and examiner have a fairly dark background so that the white pin is readily seen. The test has the double advantage that the examiner can use himself as a control while at the same time he can ensure that the patient does not move his eye.

Figure 61 shows four visual charts. Chart 1 is that of a normal subject. Chart 2 shows a central scotoma of the left eye field. This may be caused by compression of the optic nerve; by a demyelinating plaque as in disseminated sclerosis; by various poisons such as tobacco and methyl alcohol and by degenerative processes of unknown cause as, for example, Leber's optic atrophy. Chart 3 shows a bitemporal hemianopia. The hemianopia is complete with a 2 mm. target but incomplete with a 5 mm. and 10 mm. target. The upper temporal quadrants show the most severe defect and this is the usual distribution with a chiasmal compression. Chart 4 shows a homonymous hemianopia. The visual loss is almost identical in each eye. This defect is found with lesions anywhere in the optic radiations within the cerebrum. With lesions immediately posterior to the chiasma the hemianopic defects in the two eyes may be slightly different.

Eye movements

The extrinsic muscles of the eye are innervated by the 3rd, 4th and 6th nerves. When a patient complains of double vision the problem is to identify the nerve or nerves affected. Little is to be gained from a neurological point of view by distinguishing the 3rd and 4th nerves and it is sufficient to distinguish the 3rd and 6th nerves.

The 6th nerve innervates the lateral rectus muscle and it follows that if an eye cannot be deviated laterally a lesion of the 6th nerve can be inferred. A failure of movement in any other direction allows an inference of a lesion in the 3rd nerve. The problem, however, becomes more difficult when the eyes appear to be moving fully although the patient complains of diplopia. To solve the problem two rules must be remembered.

1. The two images become more separated when the target is moved in the direction of the pull of the affected muscle.
2. The false image is always displaced beyond the real image.

Figure 62 shows the situation when the internal rectus of the left eye is weak. The target is held to the right of the patient who rotates his normal right eye laterally so that the target is focused on his macula. The target, however, falls on the peripheral part of the immobile or relatively immobile left eye and as a result the false image is projected further to the right than the real image. If the target is moved further to the right the false image will be projected

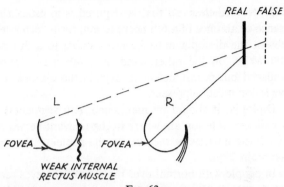

FIG. 62
Diplopia with Weakness of the Internal Rectus Muscle.

further to the right and thus will separate more from the real image. Should the patient cover his left eye the more lateral image, which is also the false one, will disappear. This diplopia is sometimes called a crossed diplopia.

Figure 63 shows the situation when the right lateral rectus is weak. In this case the target is focused on the peripheral retina of the right eye and is, therefore, projected laterally beyond the real image. When the right eye is covered the more lateral image disappears. This may be called an uncrossed diplopia.

To sum up, a diplopia produced by gaze in any direction except to right or left must be attributable to a 3rd nerve lesion. With diplopia on lateral gaze all that is required is to find which eye, when covered, extinguishes the more lateral image, for in lateral gaze one internal rectus and one lateral rectus is in action. From a knowledge of which muscle is affected, an inference of the nerve involved is easy.

When the 3rd and 6th nerves are both affected either in one eye or in both eyes the situation may be rather confusing. Nevertheless, all that is required is to establish the presence or absence of a 6th nerve lesion, for if such a lesion is absent the diplopia must be attributable to a 3rd nerve lesion while, on the other hand, if a 6th nerve lesion is established but is insufficient to explain the diplopia a 3rd nerve lesion must be present.

Diplopia, it should be mentioned, is a segmental sign and indicates a lesion anywhere in the relevant nerves from the extrinsic muscles of the eyes to the nuclei of the nerves in the brain stem.

In people with normal eyes the axes of the eyes remain parallel with all directions of gaze on a distant object. When one of the extrinsic eye muscles is weak the axes will, of course, no longer be parallel when gaze is directed in the direction of the pull of the affected muscle. The failure to maintain the parallel axes, however, although certainly related to a disorder to an extrinsic muscle, is not necessarily related to a nerve lesion. Some children develop a squint, possibly due to a refractive error of one eye, and this is

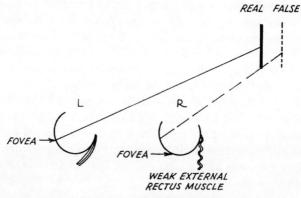

Fig. 63
Diplopia with Weakness of the External Rectus Muscle.

called a concomitant strabismus. Although the axes of the eyes are not parallel on distant gaze the relative direction of the two axes is not changed with different directions of gaze as it is with a weak muscle due to a nerve lesion.

A recent nerve lesion causing weakness of extrinsic eye muscles nearly always provokes diplopia and this is sufficient to draw a distinction between a nerve lesion and a concomitant strabismus. With a nerve lesion, however, the false image is ultimately suppressed although the rate at which this occurs is very variable. Nevertheless, the diplopia which is present in the initial stage of a nerve lesion should prevent a concomitant strabismus being wrongly diagnosed. When in doubt, careful attention to the axes of the eyes during eye movement should keep you right.

Weakness of the extrinsic muscles may be due not only to lesions of the 3rd, 4th and 6th cranial nerves but also to certain disorders of the muscles themselves which may be brought under the headings of myopathy and myasthenia gravis and to swellings of one sort or another in the orbit. These conditions produce symptoms and signs similar to those caused by nerve lesions.

Swellings in the orbit and in the retro-orbital region may cause the eye-ball to protrude and this is called proptosis. The extrinsic muscles are sometimes affected directly or secondarily due to lesions of the nerves. It is worth noting here that lesions of the optic nerve may also be produced, leading to blindness which begins as a central scotoma. Neurological lesions generally affect only one eye, whereas the exophthalmos of hyperthyroidism may affect both eyes.

Cerebrovascular lesions of the frontal lobes of the cerebrum sometimes cause both eyes to deviate involuntarily to the side of the lesion. In other words, the eyes turn away from the hemiplegic side. This deviation is usually transient and disappears in a matter of days even though the other neurological signs remain. The patient may, nevertheless, continue to be unable to deviate his eyes towards the paralysed limbs although he may be able to follow a moving object in that direction. Brain-stem lesions causing paralysis of conjugate deviation do not permit these pursuit movements. With convulsions which affect mainly the limbs of one side, the eyes and head may be rotated to the side of the affected limbs, that is, to the side opposite the frontal lobe lesion.

Pupils

It is convenient to say a few words about the pupils at this point. Reference has already been made to Argyll Robertson pupils which are small, unequal, irregular in outline and fail to respond to light although they may do so on accommodation. They should not be confused with Adie's pupils which are large and regular and react only sluggishly to strong light. Associated with these pupils there may be absent tendon jerks so that there may be confusion with tabes dorsalis if the definition of Argyll Robertson pupils is not remembered.

A 3rd nerve lesion may cause a fixed dilated pupil and this may occur alone or with weakness of the extrinsic eye muscles innervated by this nerve. It should also be mentioned that a lesion of the 3rd nerve also causes the eyelid to droop either partially or completely. With a complete 3rd nerve lesion the eye is shut and when the lid is retracted the pupil will be found to be dilated while the eye is deviated laterally under the unopposed action of the lateral rectus.

CHAPTER XXVI

THE MOTOR AND SENSORY SYSTEMS

The distinction between functional and organic signs

The distinction between functional and organic signs presents the greatest challenge a doctor has to face and is the source of his most frequent and serious errors. The definition of the terms functional and organic have already been given in Chapter XXI and need not be repeated, although it will be emphasised that the terms functional and psychogenic are not synonymous.

As an introduction the following statement deserves consideration.

In the practice of neurology functional symptoms are much more common than organic symptoms whereas organic physical signs are much more common than functional physical signs. To put the matter in another way, functional symptoms are common while functional physical signs are rare. Organic symptoms and physical signs hold an intermediate position.

In the analysis of signs it is useful to think in terms of continuous and periodic variations. Continuous and periodic mental signs have already been considered in the two chapters dealing with cerebral segmental signs and all that remains is an analysis of motor and sensory somatic signs. Before making this analysis the following general points may be made.

1. People with a functional illness are not inferior and should not be despised. You cannot avoid liking some patients and disliking others but you must not allow your

103

emotional reactions to lead you to suppose, in difficult cases, that the patients you dislike are probably functional while the patients you like are probably organic.

2. You should not place a great deal of reliance on the patient's attitude to his illness and assume that patients who complain a great deal are probably functional while patients who are more stoical are probably organic.

3. Functional signs appearing for the first time over the age of 50 years are unusual. At the same time it must be noted that a long history of functional signs does not protect a patient against organic illness.

4. The longer the history, especially if there has been no progression, the more likely are the signs to be functional.

5. Signs which show a marked response to placebos are likely to be functional.

6. Functional and organic signs are not mutually exclusive and to diagnose one is not to exclude the other.

Continuous sensory symptoms.—The quality of somatic sensory symptoms is usually of little help in distinguishing the functional from the organic. However, a picturesque and elaborate description, whether of pain or paraesthesiae, generally tips the doctor towards the diagnosis of a functional disorder although, if he is wise, he will wait until he has made a physical examination before reaching a firm conclusion. The distribution of sensory symptoms is much more useful than their quality. Symptoms which are confined to the distribution of spinal roots or peripheral nerves make an organic lesion almost certain. The converse, however, that symptoms, which are outwith the distribution of roots and nerves, are probably functional is not true. Symptoms which show a great variation in their situation are likely to be functional.

Periodic sensory symptoms.—Sensory symptoms which come and go a great deal are likely to be functional, especially if at the same time they change their situation. Two conditions, however, modify this statement. First, as stated above, symptoms which are within the distribution of roots and nerves are likely to be organic and second, symptoms which have a clear and repetitive provocation are likely to be organic. Examples of the second are the tingling of the hand in the carpal tunnel syndrome provoked by rest, the tingling or pain in an arm in cervical prolapsed disc provoked by neck movements and the tingling of the limbs with a cervical cord lesion (often disseminated sclerosis) provoked by neck flexion. Tic douloureux is a notable exception. Common periodic sensory symptoms are part of migraine but, as the term functional is at present defined, migraine is a functional condition.

Continuous motor symptoms.—Continuous motor symptoms are difficult to analyse since, unlike sensory symptoms, anatomical distributions are not readily apparent. Moreover, patients use a variety of terms, such as clumsiness, tiredness and stiffness, which leave the doctor in some doubt about the true nature of the disability being described. Nevertheless continuous symptoms suggestive of a motor defect should be suspected as organic until a physical examination reveals that they are functional.

Periodic motor symptoms.—Periodic motor symptoms, unlike sensory, are uncommon. As with sensory symptoms, clear and repetitive provocation raises the probability of an organic lesion, as for example, exercise provoking weakness or stiffness. Focal convulsions allow a sufficiently high probability inference of an organic cerebral lesion to justify special investigations. It is worth noting here that focal convulsions (without change in consciousness) associated with an abnormal EEG make an organic lesion likely.

Only one type of periodic motor symptom is almost certainly functional and this is exhlbited when a patient, in the middle of a strenuous act, feels the strength suddenly drain away from a limb.

No matter how expert a doctor may be in his analysis of symptoms and no matter how confident he may be in his conclusions he always keeps his mind open until he has completed a physical examination. Signs previously described above have all been of an organic type and it now remains to describe functional physical signs.

Functional physical motor signs.—There are a number of such signs.

1. A patient who has an LT distribution of weakness almost certainly has an organic lesion. It follows that a patient with a functional weakness must have an ST distribution although, of course, the converse is not true. An ST weakness is a most reliable functional sign provided the circumstances are appropriate. For example, when a patient's symptoms such as headache and seizures indicate that an organic lesion causing weakness (if there is such a lesion) must be LT, it follows than an ST weakness is most probably functional (unless there are multiple lesions). Similarly, ST weakness which has a hemiplegic distribution is a contradiction and strongly suggests that the weakness is functional. Lastly, when an LT sensory level in the trunk is associated with ST weakness of the legs, the signs are in conflict and indicate (if multiple or a diffuse spinal lesion are unlikely) that the weakness is functional. Remember in this connection that disseminated sclerosis does not cause ST weakness in the limbs.

2. Sometimes patients who complain of weakness respond to tests of strength in rather a peculiar way. In testing forearm extension, for example, you may find that the patient starting at the right angle position does not vary his posture although you yourself press with great or little force. In eliciting this response you should vary your pressure gradually so that the patient is unaware of the change. It would seem that patients who behave in this way suppose that their apparent inability to extend the forearm is proof of weakness but they see no inconsistency between their inability to extend the forearm against feeble resistance and their ability to maintain the forearm posture against great force. As you would suppose this type of response indicates a functional weakness.

3. Another response which has functional significance is one in which are patient's limb, during a test of strength, trembles and shakes to and fro about the starting position. It would seem that the patient supposes that his behaviour is evidence of weakness although, on the contrary, it is evidence of considerable strength. To convince yourself of this you should ask a colleague to test your forearm extension and while he exerts great force you must try to shake your arm. You will find the performance most exhausting.

4. Yet another functional response is one in which the patient exerts considerable force for a moment and then suddenly gives way. The patient, by his general demeanour, gives the impression that his effort was so great that it exhausted him. Patients with organic motor lesions do not behave in this way and when your force is excessive they gradually yield.

5. Many patients in tests of strength do not at first exert their maximum effort and you must encourage them to do so. A few patients, however, despite your exhorta-

tions, continue to make less than a maximal effort. If you are confident of this you may assume that the weakness exhibited is functional. To confirm your impression you should pay attention to other muscles. A patient who exerts his arm with much effort tightens up his shoulder muscles so that the latter may be used as evidence of the former. A good test for judging the patient's effort in hip-flexion is to place a hand under the heel of the opposite foot. Patients who make a strong effort in hip-flexion press their opposite foot strongly on the bed and you will consequently have difficulty in raising the foot with your hand. If you can raise the foot easily the inference is that the patient is not attempting hip-flexion of the opposite thigh with his maximum strength. Of course, if there is marked weakness of both legs this test should be used with caution.

6. A good indication of functional weakness is inconsistent behaviour on the part of the patient. For example, a patient who apparently cannot lift his leg from the examination couch may, a few minutes later, raise it up with obvious ease as he gets off the couch. Possibly a patient may exhibit a total paralysis of foot dorsi-flexion yet walk normally. Many such examples could be quoted. It is a good plan to watch a patient dressing and undressing and then to correlate your observations with the results of the formal motor examination.

7. A patient who claims weakness of a limb may exhibit weakness which is not only equal in the flexion and extension movements but also with regard to proximal and distal movements. A very even diffuse weakness of a limb is somewhat unusual with an organic lesion for, if the lesion is ST, proximal and distal weakness is usually not equal and flexion movements may be weaker than exten-

sion. It follows that an evenly diffuse weakness is probably functional although a firm conclusion should not be based on this sign alone. A total paralysis of a limb presents a difficult problem for the distribution of weakness in itself does not allow a distinction to be made between LT and ST lesions nor between functional and organic states. A total paralysis of one limb alone, however, is unlikely to be due to an LT lesion and if there are no organic sensory signs or reflex changes it is also unlikely to be due to an ST lesion. A complete ST paralysis, if organic, will in the course of time become associated with wasting and changes in electrical muscle reactions so that eventually a firm opinion may be given. Never explain away wasting in a paralysed limb as disuse atrophy.

Functional physical sensory signs.—The distinction between functional and organic physical sensory signs is not so clear as it is in the case of motor signs. The distribution of a functional sensory loss, of course, never coincides with spinal roots and peripheral nerves but takes the form of a glove-stocking level, a level on the trunk or a hemianaesthesia. A distinction between a functional and organic glove-stocking sensory loss may be made on the basis of the following points.

1. A glove or stocking level in one limb or in the limbs of one side is probably functional, for with polyneuritis, the usual cause of a glove-stocking loss, all the limbs are affected.

2. A glove or stocking level which coincides with joints, especially shoulder or hip, is probably functional and the probability is increased if more than one limb shows this sensory distribution.

3. A glove or stocking level which is similar for all sensory modes and for all intensities of stimulation is

probably functional. Touch sense is the only mode which can be easily varied in intensity and this is achieved by using the nylon thread described in Volume I. In an organic case the weaker the stimulus (the longer the thread) the higher is the level in the limb. In a functional case the level does not vary with different strengths of stimulus. It should be noted that in a long-standing polyneuritis, which is neither progressing nor regressing, the level may not vary with different strengths of stimulus, a state of affairs which is analogous to the visual fields of a static visual defect in which the isopters are crowded together.

In the case of sensory levels in the trunk, variations with different intensities of stimulation are not reliable and the distinction between functional and organic sensory signs has to be based on other signs. For example, a sensory level in the trunk associated with functional weakness of the legs is probably also functional.

A hemianaesthesia occurring in isolation is probably functional. When associated with other signs its interpretation depends on those signs. For example, a hemianaesthesia associated with an organic hemiplegia is best considered organic whereas a hemianaesthesia associated with segmental signs in the limbs may safely be considered functional.

As with motor signs inconsistent behaviour on the part of the patient gives a clue to a functional state. For example, a severe loss of space sense in the fingers associated with normal dexterity of the fingers (the eyes being shut) is almost certainly functional.

Conclusion.—It has already been mentioned that functional and organic signs are not mutually exclusive and it should be emphasised that they may occur in the same patient and even in the same limb. When they occur in the same limb it should not be thought that the evidence is conflicting and it should be considered that each kind of evidence allows its own valuable inference.

Pseudo-bulbar palsy

A lesion of the long motor tracts on one side produces no effect on the muscles of the tongue and throat. Bilateral long tract lesions, however, produce weakness and spasticity. This is chiefly evident in the speech which becomes slow and indistinct. The rhythm of the speech is fairly well maintained, unlike that due to a cerebellar lesion, and the term ' spastic dysarthria ' can be used as a term opposed to cerebellar dysarthria. Chewing and swallowing may also become impaired. The term ' pseudo-bulbar palsy ' is an old one and the word ' pseudo ' is meant to imply only that there is no wasting of the tongue. Patients with a pseudo-bulbar palsy may laugh or cry to a degree which is in excess of the stimulus. Laughing, too, may be provoked by sadness and crying by gladness, a state of affairs which is a source of great embarrassment to the patient. It may also cause the patient to be considered insane.

The jaw jerk may be increased with bilateral long tract motor lesions but this is a difficult jerk to assess and is best avoided.

The cranial nerves

The cranial nerves, like the spinal nerves, contain motor and sensory components and the inferences of lesions from motor and sensory signs follow the same rules. The cranial nerves may be involved as part of a polyneuritis such as infective polyneuritis and more rarely as part of a mononeuritis such as that associated with diabetes mellitus. They may also be affected by inflammatory lesions of the meninges and a meningovascular syphilis may be included in this group. In any part of their course, too, the cranial nerves may be compressed by neoplasms. At their origin in the brain-stem the cranial nerves may be affected by vascular, infective, neoplastic and demyelinating lesions. It is evident, therefore, that the cranial nerves are susceptible to many kinds of pathologies.

The diagnosis of site of lesion is influenced by two considerations. If there are LT signs it is probable that the cranial nerve lesions are near or in the brain-stem. If there are no LT signs the position of the lesion can often be inferred from the relative positions of the nerves within the skull. Thus, the 2nd, 3rd, 4th, 6th and 1st division of the 5th nerve are close together in and behind the orbit so that signs referable to several nerves of this group allow a highly probable inference of a lesion in the neighbourhood of the orbit. It is useful in this connection to remember that the medulla and pons each give rise to four cranial nerves which are easily named by counting back from 12. Furthermore, the last six cranial nerves never rise above the tentorium cerebelli while the first six nerves run along the floor of the skull towards the orbits.

Some remarks have already been made about most of the cranial nerves. The first nerve or olfactory nerve has no importance except that it is often affected by injury and rarely by a meningioma of the olfactory groove. The 8th nerve or acoustic nerve will be described by the otologist. This leaves the 9th, 10th 11th and 12th nerves still to be considered and of this group only the 10th and 12 nerves merit our attention.

The vagus or 10th nerve.—The 10th nerve has many functions but its lesions produce only a few signs of neuro-logical interest. Weakness of the palate may be produced and this is evident by the failure of the palate to rise when the patient phonates. A lesion of the nerve on one side produces a more dramatic effect, for the unaffected side of the palate rises and pulls the affected side towards the unaffected side. In assessing this deviation it is advisable to focus the attention on the raphe of the palate rather than on the uvula, for the latter may be normally a little asymmetrical. When both sides of the palate are paralysed the voice assumes a nasal quality and, on drinking, fluids may pass into the nose.

The 10th nerve also innervates the vocal cords. With a unilateral lesion there may only be some hoarseness of the voice while with bilateral lesions there may be complete aphonia and inability to cough.

The hypoglossal or 12th nerve.—When there is a lesion of one nerve, the tongue, on voluntary protrusion, bends towards the affected side. The affected side of the tongue, too, is wasted and may show fasciculations. When both nerves are affected, both sides of the tongue are wasted but the tip remains in the mid-line on protrusion provided the patient can make this movement, for the weakness may be so profound that the tongue lies in the floor of the mouth. With a unilateral lesion articulation is little affected while with bilateral lesions it may be greatly disturbed.

With bilateral long motor tract lesions there is no wasting of the tongue, although protrusion may be difficult or impossible, so that the distinction between an LT and ST lesion is easy.

The gait

The legs are commonly affected in the majority of neurological diseases and disturbances of gait are a frequent occurrence. With an LT motor lesion the leg is held stiffly at the knee and on taking a step forward the thigh is circumducted with the toes lifted only a short distance from the ground or not at all. You will remember from previous remarks that the foot is maintained in a position of plantar flexon. When only one leg is affected the patient can progress without too much difficulty but, when both legs are weak and spastic, the gait is slow and laboured. It is worth noting at this point that a patient's gait may apparently be weak and spastic although tests with the patient lying down may not be productive. This discrepancy between gait and clinical tests, a discrepancy which varies between patients, should not lead you to suspect malingering on the part of the patient.

With a cerebellar ataxia the patient lurches and reels while the movement of each leg as it moves forward is obviously incoordinate. With a sensory ataxia the patient's gait is rather deliberate, each leg being moved forward under the control of vision. This visual control may not be sufficient to prevent the patient staggering and, of course, when the visual control is removed by shutting the eyes, the staggering is greatly aggravated.

In paralysis agitans the steps are slow and shuffling with the legs maintained in a semi-flexed posture. The legs do not circumduct as they do with a spastic gait and the movements are fairly well coordinated.

Occasionally a patient is seen who walks with rather stiff knees but, unlike the spastic patient who walks mostly on the toes, keeps his feet dorsiflexed while walking on the heels. This patient, too, walks with great care and deliberation. With this appearance a functional disorder* is highly probable.

---

* The term 'functional disorder', in a neurological context, should be taken to mean functional disorder of the nervous system.

With all patients who hobble along, perhaps with the aid of sticks, it is a good plan to take their arm and walk along with them. With encouragement it may occasionally be found that the patient's walking will improve and that even when you give little physical support the patient advances fairly well. However, as soon as you allow the patient to walk on his own, his gait immediately deteriorates to its previous state. When this happens you will gain the impression that the patient has lost confidence in his walking and this suggests a functional disorder.

CHAPTER XXVII

INFERRING THE SITE OF A CEREBRAL LESION

SOME lesions are spread diffusely throughout the cerebrum while others are focal, that is to say, they are restricted to a part of the cerebrum. The terms ' diffuse ' and ' focal ' have obviously opposite meanings but their definitions are, nevertheless, difficult. If we take a lesion to mean an abnormal portion of an organ surrounded by normal tissue, then we could decide that a diffuse lesion is one which extends into both cerebral hemispheres while a focal lesion is confined to one hemisphere. Of course, each hemisphere may be the site of a focal lesion but since normal tissue separates these two lesions they are thus distinguished from one diffuse lesion. An alternative definition would be that a focal lesion occupies only a part of a hemisphere while a lesion greater than this, that is, one which is bilateral or occupies an entire hemisphere, is diffuse. The first definition, however, is more useful for our present purpose.

The following rules may be formulated.

1. The more diffuse the lesion (encephalitis, G.P.I., pre-senile dementia, Huntington's chorea, toxaemias) the more probable is psychological evidence (psychosis) although neuro-psychological evidence may also be present.

2. The more focal the lesion (neoplasm, abscess, haemorrhage, infarction) the more probable is neuro-psychological evidence and the less probable is psychological evidence.

3. From psychological evidence (psychosis) an organic lesion may be inferred with only a low probability.

4. From neuro-psychological evidence an organic lesion may be inferred with a high probability.

Rules 3 and 4 and the corollaries of 1 and 2 may be shown in a more diagrammatic way.

Focal lesion $\xleftarrow{\text{mod. p}}$ neuro-psychological evidence $\xrightarrow{\text{high p}}$ organic lesion.

Diffuse lesion $\xleftarrow{\text{high p}}$ psychological evidence $\xrightarrow{\text{low p}}$ organic lesion.

It is fortunate that some cerebral segmental signs allow high probability inferences of an organic lesion and other high probability inferences of a functional disorder. It should be noted that it is not the type of pathology which is inferred but only that the lesion is organic.

Strangely enough, most cerebral segmental signs do not allow focal inferences. The most that could be said is that the anterior portions of the cerebrum are most productive of these signs. The site of the lesion, moreover, cannot be inferred. Aphasia and focal convulsions are exceptions, the former indicating a lesion in the dominant hemisphere roughly within the area shown in Figure 64 and the latter indicating a lesion of the opposite motor areas. Agnosia and psychical seizures indicate lesions of the parietal lobes and temporal lobes respectively but whether the lesions are bilateral or not cannot be inferred.

The most frequent focal signs are really a combination of a cerebral segmental sign and an LT sign. It should perhaps be emphasised that a focal sign is one from which a focal lesion can be inferred. The long motor and sensory tracts have a fairly circumscribed pathway through the cerebrum and if, on the basis of a cerebral segmental sign it

117

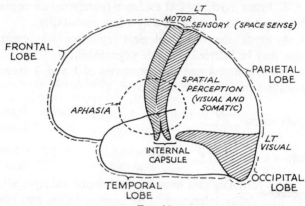

FIG. 64

The Inference of the Site of a Cerebral Lesion.

Frontal Lobe. Contralateral LT motor signs. Contralateral convulsions. Aphasia. Dementia. Amnesia.

Parietal Lobe. Contralateral sensory signs. Spatial agnosia. Contralateral hemianopia. Somato-sensory seizures. Aphasia. Dementia. Amnesia.

Temporal Lobe. Contralateral hemianopia. Contralateral LT motor signs. Psychical seizures. Aphasia. Dementia. Amnesia.

Occipital Lobe. Contralateral hemianopia.

Aphasia is caused by a lesion of the dominant hemisphere. The degree of dementia and amnesia is related to the quantity of cerebrum disturbed rather than to the site of the lesion. Generalised convulsions may be caused by lesions anywhere in the cerebrum.

can be inferred that there is a cerebral lesion, then the position of the lesion can be inferred from the LT sign. Sometimes an LT sign is referred to as a focal cerebral sign but in this event it is implied that a cerebral segmental sign is also present. An example of this combination of signs will make the matter clear. A patient who exhibits dementia and has a left hemiplegia, has a focal lesion in the right cerebral hemisphere somewhere between the motor cortex and the

THE INFERENCE OF CEREBRAL LESIONS FROM
CLINICAL EVIDENCE

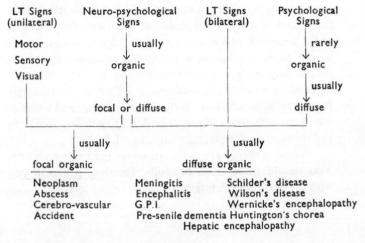

FIG. 65

internal capsule. At this point it should be mentioned that in the internal capsule the motor fibres are bunched together while in the motor cortex they are spread out. You will remember that the body is represented upside-down in the motor cortex and that the hand and face areas are close together in the lower part of the precentral gyrus while the leg area is in the upper part on the medial aspect of the hemisphere. Lesions in the motor cortex may, therefore, pick out parts of the body and, while this is fortunate from the point of view of localisation of lesions, it is unfortunate from the point of view of identifying signs, for the LT distribution of weakness may be obscured. For example, a

119

lesion in the hand area may give a severe isolated weakness of the hand, a distribution which is really of a segmental type. You should be on the look-out for this. As a rule the presence of cerebral segmental signs or facial weakness will keep you right. This is a convenient point to mention that a rapid and severe LT weakness of the face often includes slight weakness of eye closure. This appearance is similar to the recovery stage of a severe ST weakness and if the patient does not give a good history you may have difficulty in deciding whether the weakness is LT or ST. Fortunately hand weakness, which is nearly always present, and aphasia, which is sometimes present, will help you to decide in certain cases that the facial weakness is LT.

These remarks are summarised in Figures 64 and 65. You should study them carefully, for they will help you with the next three chapters.

CHAPTER XXVIII

A REVIEW OF THE NEUROLOGICAL EXAMINATION*

SINCE the number of examination techniques already described is sufficient for a fairly complete neurological examination, it is essential that we should now arrange the tests in some convenient order. Before doing so it is important to emphasise that you must get into the habit of making inferences and changing probabilities at every step of the examination, for it is only by so doing that you will make modifications in your routine examination to suit the individual patient. The worst kind of examination is one in which the clinician relentlessly and blindly pursues a complex and routine battery of tests without considering inferences until he has accumulated a large quantity of evidence. The fault in this method is that many tests are needlessly performed, while some important tests are omitted.

The best approach to a neurological problem is to divide the examination into four phases.

Phase 1

This phase consists of history-taking. We are not concerned at the moment with the method of history-taking but rather with the evidence which is thereby obtained. It has already been remarked that history-taking should be directed towards constructing a satisfactory sign-time graph but history-taking is also important in other respects, for the

---

* The student is advised to read this chapter again when subsequent chapters have been assimilated.

symptoms elicited may be segmental signs and furthermore, during history-taking, you may observe neuro-psychological signs such as inattention, dementia, amnesia and aphasia. It, of course, goes without saying that, if any of these signs are severe or if the patient is unconscious, you are obliged to turn to friends and relations for the history of the patient's illness.

At the end of this phase you should pause and make two decisions. First, whether the history is adequate, for, if not, you must amplify it by accounts given by witnesses. And second, you should decide whether neuro-psychological signs are present or absent. If you have any doubts, you should make a mental note to return to the problem in Phase 3. If Phase 1 has gone well you should feel fairly confident whether you are dealing with an organic or functional illness and, in the case of the former, you should have singled out the types which are most probable.

Phase 2

This phase consists of a routine physical examination which should be applied to every patient as part of a general medical examination. You should practise the tests on every patient you examine and, in doing so, you should aim at a fast and smooth performance. Five minutes are ample for the entire phase. The order of testing is as follows.

1. The fundi and eye movements are examined. The pupils, nystagmus, voluntary eye movements and diplopia should be noted.
2. A routine motor examination is performed.
3. A routine sensory examination is performed.
4. The coordination of arm movements is tested (the finger-nose test). If the patient is ambulant the gait can be tested later. Otherwise, the heel-knee test

may be done. It may be noted, however, that, in a bed ridden patient suffering from a nervous disease, this test is, as a rule, superfluous since there is a multitude of other signs.

You will notice that, apart from the eye tests, this phase of the examination consists of LT tests although during the motor and sensory examination it may become apparent that the signs are of an ST type. Special ST motor tests, however, should not be done and no attempt should be made to demonstrate sensory levels.

In the majority of patients you examine, Phase 2 will give negative results and, when there are no neurological symptoms, the neurological examination may be considered to be completed.

Phase 3

In Phase 3 the aim is to demonstrate mainly ST signs. You should not, of course, attempt to look for ST signs everywhere and you have therefore to choose one level of the nervous system for your attack. The best way of thinking about the problem is to divide lesions into those which are cranial and those which are extracranial,* that is, in the spinal cord or peripheral nerves. Many signs point to a cranial site and these are psychological signs, neuropsychological signs, headache, seizures, cranial nerve signs (including papilloedema), weakness of the face and limbs of one side, dysarthria and difficulty in chewing and swallowing. If present, these signs should be discovered during Phases 1 and 2 of the examination and all that remains to be done in Phase 3 is to check doubtful signs, to perform tests for neuro-psychological signs in detail if this seems

---

* There are, of course, a few diseases which produce signs in both situations.

necessary and to examine the visual fields first by confrontation and later on the Bjerrum screen. It will be mentioned later that intracranial lesions may be divided into those above the tentorium cerebelli and those below and, when the latter site is suspected, all cranial nerves, except the first two, should be carefully tested.

In the absence of signs enumerated above, the search for ST signs must be directed towards the limbs and trunk. If a pain loss has been discovered in Phase 2 it is advisable, in Phase 3, to proceed immediately to the demonstration of sensory levels. Once this is completed it is a simple matter to decide where to look for ST motor signs. The demonstration of levels with space sense, vibration sense or touch sense should be delayed (if it need be done at all) until the motor examination is completed and the position of the lesion identified with some confidence.

With regard to motor signs the routine examination of Phase 2 is sufficient to identify them as LT or ST or a mixture of both. When there is a mixture of motor signs the usual situation is that LT signs are found in the legs while ST signs or both ST and LT signs are found in the arms. Should the signs be purely of an ST type the routine examination of Phase 2 makes it evident whether such signs are distributed in all the limbs or only in some, and whether they are more marked distally or proximally. With this knowledge it is easy to plan further motor and sensory examinations for, by this stage, you should be beginning to think of certain diseases.

When the motor signs are purely of an LT type the problem becomes a little difficult. With bilateral signs the probability of a cerebral or brain-stem lesion is low and the probability of a spinal lesion high. With the first two the probability is low when cerebral segmental signs and cranial nerve signs respectively are absent, while the probability is considerably raised when these signs are present. LT motor signs confined to the legs are of no value in determining the site of a lesion in the pyramidal tracts but signs in the arms indicate that the lesion is in the cervical cord or higher; and signs in the face indicate that the lesion is in the pons or higher. The ST motor and sensory examination can, therefore, be suitably limited when the face or arm is involved.

Isolated cerebellar signs present a most difficult problem for, although a lesion of the central nervous system is most probable, the level of the lesion is not easily established. Of course, a cerebellar dysarthria or a truncal ataxia indicates that the cerebellum itself is the seat of a lesion but otherwise there is no way of inferring the level of the lesion.

We have now to face the difficult problem of what to do when a patient with neurological symptoms exhibits no neurological signs during Phases 1 and 2 of the examination. The trouble is that there is a large variety of neurological symptoms which, in the majority of patients, have no organic cause and consequently, when presented with these symptoms, there is the temptation to omit an ST examination. This temptation should be resisted in the early years of your professional life although in later years experience may justify a type of examination which, to the novice, may seem careless and superficial. The method of approach with patients who complain of weakness or other symptoms referable to the motor system is to inquire about the site of the weakness or about the particular movements which are found difficult and then to apply an ST motor examination to that area. With patients who complain of general weakness, although this has probably no neurological significance provided the Phase 2 examination is negative, it is advisable to check the shoulder, pelvic and trunk muscles. The easiest method of testing the last is to ask the patient to rise from a supine position without using the arms. This test is useful in patients with myopathy and myasthenia gravis. In the same way, patients complaining of sensory symptoms should be asked to specify the site of their symptoms and, if they can do this with some precision, an ST motor and sensory examination may be applied to a limited area.

Phase 4

This phase consists of special investigations. Special investigations may be divided into two types. The first includes blood chemical and cellular analysis (including the ESR), urine chemical analysis, serological tests such as the WR, EEGs and straight X-rays. These tests may be applied at out-patient departments on patients broadly selected. The second type, which should be reserved for a narrowly selected group of in-patients, includes lumbar puncture and a variety of neuro-radiological procedures. All these tests, it should be noted, follow the tests of the first three phases and should never be allowed to substitute for these tests.

By the end of Phase 3 you should have lowered the probability of all but one or two diseases to a negligible level. Reference has already been made to negligible and working probabilities and it has been indicated that the numerical probabilities indicated by the terms ' negligible ' and ' working ' are different for the general practitioner and the specialist. Clearly a working level may be fairly low when the general practitioner is considering referring a patient to a specialist or when he is considering the first type of special investigations enumerated above (these tests should be within the ambit of the general practitioner). But a working probability should have a fairly high numerical level when lumbar puncture and special neuro-radiological techniques are being considered by the specialist.

Special investigations, particularly of the second type, should only be instituted when they are capable of altering the probabilities of the one or two diseases inferred with a working level at the end of Phase 3 and when the changes in the probabilities will materially affect the management of a case with regard to therapy and the giving of a prognosis. You will, of course, have noticed that the terms ' fairly high ' and ' fairly low probabilities ' have been used above in a very loose sort of way but it is impossible to use them otherwise for clinicians differ a great deal among themselves in respect of the investigations which, in a particular patient, should be judged worthwhile. When you have worked in several units you will come to realise that some clinicians order special investigations in great numbers while others order them only rarely. There is no question of laying down rules, for the individual clinician must be given complete freedom to go his own way. Some objection to indiscriminate investigation may perhaps be raised when the investigations ordered by one clinician unnecessarily raise the cost of the medical services or make unnecessary work for another clinician.

As you read descriptions of diseases you should think of the special investigations which are relevant to each. By and large, special neuro-radiological procedures are confined to the investigation of compressive lesions and vascular disorders while CSF examination is confined to the investigation of infections, spinal compression and subarachnoid haemorrhage. Blood and urine tests, with the exception of the ESR, are useful only in the investigation of various blood, metabolic and toxic disorders. The EEG is a special case and a later chapter is devoted to it.

Headaches and seizures present a common problem with regard to special investigations. When they are associated with physical signs, special investigations can be planned with confidence but, when they occur in isolation, the problem may be most difficult. Headaches and seizures are common effects of many kinds of intracranial pathology although, on the other hand, they are frequently in the nature of functional disorders of the nervous system. The clinician's dilemma is therefore easily understood. Straight X-rays and EEGs may, of course, be used (although they are only occasionally helpful) as a first line of investigation on fairly large numbers of patients but obviously special neuro-radiological procedures can be performed on only a few. Fortunately the selection of the few may safely be left to the specialist and need not concern us further although it may be added that the general rule is that special neuro-radiological procedures are not performed unless the patient exhibits physical signs or is severely disabled.*

The necessity for special investigations in a particular patient is not the only problem to be faced in Phase 4, for there is also the problem of the speed with which special investigations should be brought into play. It may be accepted as a rule that a patient demands urgent investigation when the disease under consideration is one which

puts the patient in immediate danger,

or requires early treatment if recovery is not to be jeopardised,

or is evolving rapidly.

* Seizures beginning in, or confined to, one side offer, in themselves some justification for neuro-radiology. Reference should be made to the chapter on EEGs.

On the basis of these criteria it follows that acute infective and severe compressive lesions, intracranial and spinal, must be treated as emergencies. When none of these criteria are present it is safe to postpone special investigation.

Conclusion

This review of the neurological examination requires a good deal of digestion. Phases 1 and 2, being part of a routine general medical examination, are quickly learned. Phases 3 and 4, being more specialised, are more difficult to understand since there is less opportunity for practising them. The important lesson contained in the review is that throughout the examination you must have your wits about you and you must keep thinking. If you learn this lesson well you will find diagnostic neurology a fairly simple matter. Otherwise you will constantly be in trouble.

It has previously been stated that there are two kinds of correlative propositions in clinical medicine. In one, pathology is given as an inference and, in the other, signs are given as inferences. It is the second kind which you will find in descriptions of diseases in textbooks. At the bed-side, during the four phases of the examination, you must try to translate textbook propositions into ones which have pathology as an inference. As you gain experience you should also practise translating bed-side propositions into textbook ones. If you doubt the wisdom of this, observe some of your contemporaries. Some, you will find, are excellent diagnosticians and yet cannot pass examinations in which descriptions of diseases are requested while others, who have an encyclopaedic knowledge of diseases, are poor diagnosticians. You must practise with both kinds of propositions until you feel at ease with either. But always remember that the real skill in medicine is in discovering evidence and knowing what sort of evidence to look for.

CHAPTER XXIX

FOCAL INTRACRANIAL LESIONS

Intracranial neoplasms

THE intracranial cavity is divided into two compartments by the tentorium cerebelli. This division is of clinical importance and you should perhaps refresh your memory of it by referring to an anatomy book. Neoplasms above the tentorium are referred to as supratentorial neoplasms. The cavity below the tentorium is often called the posterior fossa. The cerebrum occupies the supratentorial cavity and the cerebellum and brainstem the posterior fossa. As you would expect, the clinical evidence of neoplasms on either side of the tentorium is very different.

There are many kinds of primary intracranial neoplasms* but they can be divided into two main types called infiltrative and non-infiltrative. These types can also be called malignant and benign respectively although it should be remembered that primary malignant neoplasms of the nervous system do not give rise to blood-borne metastasis.

The infiltrative neoplasms of the nervous system are called gliomata. There are many varieties, the most important being spongioblastoma multiforme which is a rapidly growing neoplasm of the cerebrum of adults;

* The student should refer to a textbook of pathology for a complete list of intracranial neoplasms.

astrocytoma which is a slow growing neoplasm of the cerebrum of adults and of the cerebellum of children; medulloblastoma and ependymoma which grow in the region of the 4th ventricle of children, the former being fast growing and the latter slow.

There are also several varieties of benign neoplasms, the most important being meningioma, acoustic neurofibroma, angioma and pituitary adenoma. All these benign neoplasms arise externally to the central nervous system although by virtue of their growth they may ultimately push their way into cerebral and brainstem substance.

The cerebrum and cerebellum are common sites of secondary carcinoma. Secondary hypernephroma and melanoma are rare.

Neoplasms produce their effects in three ways.

1. By compression and traction of nervous tissue nearby and at a distance.
2. By the local destruction of nervous tissue by neoplastic cells.
3. By the production of toxins.

The pressure effects of neoplasms.—Neoplasms produce their pressure effects in two ways. They may compress tissues immediately adjacent, causing their death perhaps by anoxia or, if they are large, they may distort the intracranial structures even at a distance. The latter has probably little effect on the brain substance provided it slowly develops but traction on the meninges, cranial nerves and blood vessels may produce pain and loss of function. The local compressive effects on the cerebrum are minimal unless the neo-plasm is very large or unless the neoplasm is in such a position that a loss of nervous tissue readily produces signs and symptoms.

The second way in which a neoplasm produces pressure effects is by interference with the circulation of CSF through the ventricular system. Should a neoplasm block this circulation the ventricular system proximally expands to accommodate the continuous production of CSF by the choroid plexus. This ven-tricular expansion is capable of compressing all intra-cranial structures. There are several important points about this method of producing pressure. A small neoplasm may block the ventricular system in the region of the 3rd and 4th ventricles and of the aqueduct which connects them and, as a result, the lateral ven-tricles may enlarge greatly, producing effects which seem, at first sight, out of proportion to the size of the neoplasm. It follows, too, that a small neoplasm below the tentorium may produce pressure effects above. Lastly, the increasing pressure effect of the expanding lateral ventricles may force the cerebral structures through the notch in the tentorium cerebelli where a rise of pressure further impedes the circulation of the CSF. There is thus set into operation a vicious circle in which the effect increases the cause. The plugging of the notch of the tentorium by the cerebral struc-tures (the so-called coning) will only occur if the pres-sure above the tentorium is substantially above that below the tentorium. If the pressure above and below the tentorium is raised considerably the effect may be to push the cerebellum into the foramen magnum, again introducing a vicious circle of pressure effects.

The expansion of the ventricular system may be called a hydrocephalus. This expansion may be the result of a block in the CSF circulation as already indicated or an atrophy of the cerebrum. In the present context we are only considering the hydrocephalus produced by pressure.

For the moment we will ignore the pressure effects immediately adjacent to a neoplasm and consider only the effects of a general rise of intracranial pressure. Headache, which is produced by the compression and traction of extra-cerebral tissues, has an aching quality and, if severe, may be said to have a bursting quality. It may be general or focal but is rarely confined to a small area of the head, small enough that is, for the patient to point to it with one finger. It may be paroxysmal in the early stages but as the pressure increases it becomes continuous although possibly varying in severity. This headache is often associated with vomiting which may not be accompanied by nausea. It may be increased by coughing and stooping.

Swelling of the optic disks is good evidence of an increase of intracranial pressure. This swelling, called papilloedema, is easily identified when severe but mild degrees may be difficult to diagnose. Since the clinician looks down on the swelling with his opthalmoscope it is only possible to infer a swelling from the different lenses required to bring the retina and disk into focus.

This is too difficult a technique for the beginner. The best way of identifying papilloedema is to direct the attention to the edge of the disk. In papilloedema the swelling causes the vessels to be obscured in this part of their course. The edge of the disk should otherwise be ignored for blurring of the margin is not necessarily indicative of swelling. With papilloedema the veins become swollen although this as an isolated sign is not very reliable evidence of increased intracranial pressure. Lastly, haemorrhages and exudates may be found in the fundus. The appearance of the disks so far described may be found with focal lesions of the optic nerve. Such lesions may be a product of vascular hypertension which you will learn about elsewhere. From a neurological point of view an important lesion is a plaque of demyelination in the optic nerve. If this is behind the disk (the so-called retro-orbital neuritis) there may be no visible effects except pallor of the disk at a later stage, but should the disk be involved some swelling may be apparent. This swelling never reaches the severe degrees of papilloedema although it is difficult to distinguish from the milder degrees of the latter. The distinction must be made on the disturbance of vision for with papilloedema there may either be no visual defect or, if there is, the defect is in the peripheral parts of the fields. With the optic neuritis of disseminated sclerosis, on the other hand, there is always a defect of vision in the central part of the field. The patient, it should be noted, is acutely aware of a central scotoma but may be totally unaware of a peripheral defect.

It is unfortunate that papilloedema produces only a peripheral loss of vision in its early stages for a patient is generally content that his vision is intact if he can see to read. The loss of peripheral vision with papilloedema may therefore advance steadily without the patient or clinician being aware of it unless, of course, the latter takes the trouble to chart the visual fields. In a late stage of severe papilloedema, and it is only with severe papilloedema that sight is endangered, the vision may be restricted to the centre of the fields and this may be extinguished within a period of hours. The tragedy of this situation is that the blindness is nearly always bilateral, for papilloedema is nearly always bilateral, and that a relief of intracranial pressure although quickly executed will not restore vision. Some patients, for a few days before the final and complete loss of vision, complain that their vision fades for a few moments at a time. This symptom associated with severe papilloedema is an ominous sign.

It is obviously advisable, when you have diagnosed papilloedema, to refer the patient to a neurosurgeon without delay. If you have any doubts about the diagnosis of papilloedema do not hesitate to consult a more experienced clinician.

It is advisable, if you are a male, to have your colour vision tested for if you have a defect you may have difficulty in the use of the ophthalmoscope. If you are aware that you have a defect of colour vision you will no doubt take extra care with difficult cases.

Patients with a pressure hydrocephalus may appear mentally dull. This dullness is really in the nature of inattention for if a patient is vigorously roused he will be found not to be demented unless of course the neoplasm is producing local destructive effects on the cerebrum. Thus a patient with a cerebellar neoplasm may appear at first sight to be demented until it is demonstrated that he is only inattentive. If this point is not emphasised a frontal neoplasm and a cerebellar neoplasm may not be clearly distinguished. It is to be expected that as the pressure rises the mental dullness will increase and eventually the patient will become unconscious. This latter event is probably always associated with tentorial and foramen magnum coning. With the former the pupils may be seen to dilate so that this sign, associated with papilloedema and stupor, makes the situation unpleasantly clear to the clinician.

The evolution of raised intracranial pressure is variable. In most cases it must be admitted that the evolution is fairly even although the speed of evolution will obviously depend on the underlying pathology. A slow evolution, however, may become speeded up when the vicious circle already mentioned makes its appearance. In a few patients the block of the CSF circulation may be intermittent so that the signs of pressure may come and go. With a benign neoplasm (colloid cyst) of the 3rd ventricle the block may occur abruptly producing sudden severe headache and possibly loss of consciousness.

It must be stated before leaving the subject of increased pressure that pathologies other than neoplasms may produce a block. Thus abscesses, granulo-mata and meningitis may produce all the pressure effects so far described under neoplasms. Pressure signs, like all other signs, do not allow inferences of types of lesion. Nevertheless, since neoplasms are the commonest cause of a pressure hydrocephalus, the signs of the latter allow a high probability inference of an intracranial neoplasm.

Otitic hydrocephalus, a condition for which no cause is known, consists of a marked rise of intracranial pressure producing the signs already described. There are no other neurological signs except perhaps a 6th nerve palsy. A 6th nerve palsy may be caused by a raised intracranial pressure whatever the underlying pathology. In these circumstances it is said to be a false localising sign for the nerve affected is usually on the opposite side to the neoplasm responsible for the rise in pressure. With a pressure hydrocephalus both nerves may be affected.

Otitic hydrocephalus may last for several months and then subside spontaneously. It presents no danger to life but severe papilloedema may lead to blindness if the pressure is not relieved. A confident diagnosis can only be based on ventriculography which will be described later.

The local destructive effects of neoplasms.—In-filtrative neoplasms may cause the death of nervous tissue which lies in their path and this may be considered as a local toxic effect. We have now to consider the effects of this local destruction. However, these effects are no different from those produced by the death of nervous tissue caused by near and distant compression and traction and so the following remarks will include all the effects of neoplasms other than those caused by a pressure hydrocephalus.

Supratentorial neoplasms.—For the moment we will consider only cerebral neoplasms. The signs produced are related, of course, to the site of the neoplasm and this correlation has previously been discussed in some detail. At present it is necessary to concentrate our attention on the evolution of signs which allow an inference of a neoplasm. On the whole the evolution of clinical evidence of a neoplasm is fairly even although the rate is variable. Thus the clinical picture of a spongioblastoma evolves in a few weeks or months, while that of an astrocytoma and meningioma may take several years. While it is true that signs evolving over a period of years must be attributable to a slow lesion, a rapid evolution does not necessarily indicate a fast lesion. For example, a slowly growing neoplasm may produce no signs for a long time and then, when a certain stage is reached, give rise to an acute picture. You can suppose, if you want an explanation for this, that compensatory mechanisms offset the effects of a slowly growing neoplasm until a point is reached where a small increase in size causes the compensatory mechanism to break down. Apart from this the development of a hydrocephalus may obscure the evolution of a slowly growing neoplasm. Another difficulty, although admittedly a rare one, is that once a patient is admitted to hospital the signs and symptoms may diminish, due perhaps to an improvement in the general condition of the patient attributable to nursing care and adequate nutrition and fluid intake.

When the condition evolves over a matter of months the inference of a neoplasm may be made with a fairly high probability but when it evolves over days or is extended over years the probability is not so high. With reference to the former a vascular lesion or acute infective condition must be considered as a possibility and with reference to the latter a degenerative condition must be considered.

In view of these remarks it would appear that, in some cases, a diagnosis of neoplasm cannot be made with confidence on the basis of a bedside examination and consequently neuro-radiological and pathological examinations must be performed.

There are several kinds of pituitary adenomata but it is only the chromophobe and eosinophil type which become sufficiently large to produce neurological signs. A pituitary neoplasm grows in relation to the optic chiasma so that a bitemporal hemianopia is produced. The neoplasm grows slowly over months and years causing at first only headache and later a visual defect in the upper temporal fields. The visual defect progresses until a complete bitemporal hemianopia is evident and then later the nasal fields are affected until the vision in one or both eyes is destroyed. When the neoplasm becomes very large the 3rd ventricle may be compressed and a pressure hydrocephalus produced.

It should be noted, however, that the compression of the chiasma and optic nerves prevents the development of papilloedema.

The optic disks throughout either have a normal appearance or assume a pale, almost white, appearance. This pale appearance is produced by compression of the optic nerves no matter the pathology and also by any lesion which produces death of the nervous tissue of the nerve. It is often said that atrophy of the optic nerve can be inferred from pallor of the disk but the truth is that pallor without any visual defect, past or present, has doubtful significance. It is worth noting here that severe papilloedema which has proceeded to total blindness gradually subsides leaving behind a pale disk.

A somewhat similar picture to that of a pituitary adenoma may be produced by a neoplasm called a craniopharyngioma which grows above the chiasma. This, however, occurs mainly in children, whereas the pituitary tumour is confined to adults.

Posterior fossa neoplasms.—The posterior fossa contains the cerebellum, brain-stem and the origins of the cranial nerves except the first two. These structures are compact and are, as it were, crowded together, with the result that a neoplasm of one often causes a disturbance of the others. Moreover, the aqueduct and 4th ventricle are readily blocked and consequently a pressure hydrocephalus quickly arises and may overshadow the local effects of neoplasms on nervous tissue.

The signs of a pressure hydrocephalus and LT motor and sensory signs occurring in isolation do not allow a high probability inference of a posterior fossa neoplasm. However, a combination of papilloedema and *bilateral* LT signs raises the probability to a high level. The reason is that papilloedema points to an intracranial lesion and within the skull it is frequently in the brain-stem, and less commonly in the cerebrum, that a *single* neoplasm will produce bilateral signs.

Cranial nerve signs in isolation do not allow a high probability inference of a posterior fossa lesion since these nerves have quite a long course outside the fossa. Cerebellar signs, too, with the exception of a cerebellar dysarthria, being LT signs, do not allow high probability inferences of a posterior fossa lesion. However, a combination of cerebellar signs with cranial nerve signs clearly puts the lesion in the posterior fossa and to this it may be added that a combination of cerebellar signs* with papilloedema allows the same inference.

The first six cranial nerves have at least part of their course above the tentorium so that lesions of these nerves combined with papilloedema do not necessarily point to a posterior fossa neoplasm. On the other hand, the last six cranial nerves do not travel above the tentorium and it follows that lesions of these nerves combined with papilloedema indicate a posterior fossa lesion with a very high probability.

* A frontal lobe neoplasm will occasionally produce an inco-ordination of movement indistinguishable from a cerebellar ataxia.

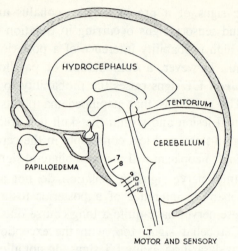

FIG. 66

The Inference of a Posterior Fossa Lesion.
Combinations of Signs Giving Highly Probable Inferences of a Posterior Fossa Lesion.
A. Papilloedema and cerebellar signs.
B. Papilloedema and bilateral LT motor and sensory signs.
This combination occurs occasionally with cerebral lesions.
C. Papilloedema and signs referable to any of the last six cranial nerves.
D. Cerebellar signs and signs referable to any of the cranial nerves.
E. LT motor and sensory signs and signs referable to the last six cranial nerves.

You will see from the above remarks that an inference of a posterior fossa lesion is based on combinations of signs. At first you may find this a little confusing but if you refer to Figure 66 and think about the problem for a little the difficulties will disappear. Papilloedema raises the probability of a neoplasm but without this sign the inference of type of pathology must of course rest on the evolution of signs. In all cases neuro-radiological examinations are required to raise the probabilities to a very high level.

The order of appearance of signs of posterior fossa neoplasms is partly determined by the site of origin of the neoplasms. Thus a cerebellar neoplasm will usually first present with cerebellar signs to be followed by papilloedema, LT signs and cranial nerve signs. On the other hand, a brain-stem neoplasm may present with LT signs or cranial nerve signs. Nevertheless it must be remembered that the order of appearance of signs is variable. There is one neoplasm which gives a fairly characteristic evolution and this is an acoustic neurofibroma. The neurofibroma arises from the 8th nerve as it enters the internal acoustic meatus. Deafness is an early sign. So far nothing has been said about hearing for you will learn a good deal about this from the otologist. Nystagmus is common since the vestibular component of the 8th nerve is affected. The 7th and 8th nerves run in close proximity in the posterior fossa and consequently a facial palsy readily occurs. This is a segmental type of weakness but has a much slower evolution than Bell's palsy. To sum up, deafness, nystagmus and facial palsy in combination raise the probability of an acoustic neurofibroma considerably. As the neoplasm enlarges it produces cerebellar signs and possibly 5th nerve signs on the same side. Eventually a pressure hydrocephalus develops with its attendant signs. In the late stages LT motor and sensory signs may appear although as a rule they are minimal and overshadowed by the other signs. It should perhaps be emphasised that patients with an acoustic neurofibroma rarely have vertigo although they commonly have cerebellar ataxia. The clinical picture which has been described is of course a reflection of the site of the neoplasm and not of its type. The site, sometimes referred to as the cerebellopontine angle, may be occupied by a meningioma or secondary carcinoma and consequently the clinical picture may be roughly similar.

The toxic effects of neoplasms.—If brain neoplasms such as meningiomata and neurofibromata cause death, they do so by their pressure effects. Gliomata and carcinomata, on the other hand, sometimes produce death without much pressure change and indeed without much destruction of tissue. It seems probable, therefore, that these malignant neoplasms produce toxins. There is some evidence of this during life for patients often look ill and this appearance seems to be unrelated to pain or neurological disability. It is impossible to describe the appearance of a patient who has a malignant neoplasm and you should therefore make your own observations.

This appearance of a patient, which can only be referred to as looking ill, is very important clinically for it may precede other evidence of disease or may occur when other evidence is minimal. A patient, for example, may present with headache which on analysis does not allow a high probability inference of an organic lesion and yet his appearance may arouse your suspicions of a malignant neoplasm. It should perhaps be emphasised that the ill look which we are at present considering is different from that exhibited by a patient who has an infection or who is distressed with pain or lack of sleep. Patients with malignant neoplasm may feel tired and listless and may lose weight. Some degree of apathy may also be present although with intracranial neoplasms this may in part be attributable to the local effects on the cerebrum.

Abscess

A patient with an intracranial abscess often has the constitutional signs and symptoms of an infection. A patient with an acute infection feels ill and by this we mean that he feels listless. To this symptom may be added headache, nausea, anorexia and vomiting. The apathy, which is evident when an attempt is made to converse with the patient, is also betrayed by his lack of facial expression, by the toneless appearance of his face and by the heaviness of his eyelids. When the toxaemia is severe the level of consciousness may deteriorate until the patient becomes moribund.

The commonest sign of infection is, of course, a rise in temperature and as a rule this is associated with tachycardia. The skin may be flushed and moist while, with a fluctuating temperature, shivering may be evident. A rise in the ESR is usually associated with fever whatever the cause but a leucocytosis is only to be expected with pyogenic infections.

These constitutional signs and symptoms are very important with regard to intracranial abscesses for on the one hand they may be helpful diagnostically and on the other they may be misleading. First, when the clinical evidence leads you to infer an intracranial lesion the constitutional signs considerably increase the probability of an intracranial infection. Second, the apathy, headache and vomiting which is a product of toxaemia may lead you to suspect an intracranial lesion even when none is present. The way out of the difficulty is to estimate the balance of constitutional signs. Thus with a severe toxaemia the degree of apathy corresponds with the degree of other constitutional signs, while with an intracranial infection the apathy is much in excess of the other signs. The explanation probably is that the rise of intracranial pressure produced by intracranial infection increases the apathy which is directly due to toxaemia. Furthermore, the local effects of infection on nervous tissue may aggravate this apathy. One other point deserves mention. With a rise of intracranial pressure the pulse rate may become slowed. In non-infective conditions this slowing, which is rarely marked, has little diagnostic value but in intracranial infections the absence of the expected tachycardia may arouse your suspicions of an intracranial abscess.

The majority of brain abscesses occur in the temporal lobes and cerebellar hemispheres and these sites are determined by the proximity of the mastoid air cells which become infected secondarily to an otitis media. Healthy ears therefore reduce the probability of an abscess while a purulent discharge increases it. A frontal lobe abscess is relatively uncommon and is secondary to an infected frontal sinus. Abscesses may be multiple when the infection is blood-borne from a distant source such as bronchiectasis. These abscesses may remain fairly small and this, with their multiplicity, may produce a somewhat confused clinical picture.

The association of cerebral segmental signs (with or without LT signs) with the constitutional signs of infection make the inference of a cerebral abscess highly probable. You should note that neuro-psychological signs do not serve to distinguish abscess from encephalitis and meningitis but the addition of a hemiplegia, aphasia or hemianopia makes a cerebral abscess much more probable and it may be added that cerebellar ataxia or nystagmus makes a cerebellar abscess probable. It can be taken as a rule that when a cerebral abscess produces fairly marked focal signs there will be an impairment of consciousness; or to put it another way, a patient who is fully attentive and conscious and has substantial focal cerebral signs is unlikely to have a cerebral abscess. It should be noted that when a patient is put on antibiotic drugs in the early stage of the illness those statements are no longer valid. Moreover, the constitutional signs upon which so much emphasis has been placed may disappear although the abscess continues to exert its effect upon the brain.

The evolution of an intracranial abscess is rather variable and this no doubt is a reflection of the nature of the infecting organism and the patient's ability to combat it. When the organism is virulent the neurological picture may evolve in a few hours but otherwise the evolution may extend over days or weeks. However, the longer the period over which progression is extended the less likely is an abscess. As in the case of neoplasms the development of a pressure hydrocephalus and the appearance of signs and symptoms usually associated with it may at any point aggravate the patient's condition.

An intracranial abscess nearly always ends in death if left untreated and even with neurosurgical measures and the use of antibiotics the mortality approaches 50 per cent. The prognosis of disability is impossible to give since it depends so much on the diagnostic and therapeutic skill of the clinician.

Vascular disorders

Structural changes in the walls of arteries form the basis of most vascular disorders. Such changes may lead to a diminution of the volume of blood circulating or to a rupture of the vessel. Sometimes the artery wall may swell up to form an aneurysm and in addition to the effects produced by a block or a burst there may be signs produced by the compression of nervous tissue.

To begin with we will confine ourselves to the blocking and bursting of arteries, the so-called cerebrovascular accidents. Clinically the effects are similar in the majority of cases. Blockage of an artery may be caused by a blood clot forming *in situ* or by a clot, now called an embolism, carried from a distant source. The blockage of an artery causes an anoxia of nervous tissue and the necrosis of tissue which follows is called an infarction.* It should be remembered that it is anoxia that kills tissue and with this in mind it will be realised that a vessel partially blocked by atheroma can be a co-existent cause of anoxia if the general circulation fails as a result of shock, haemorrhage or cardiac failure.

The diagnosis of cerebrovascular accidents.—Cerebral infarction and haemorrhage are rare in young people and it is not until the age of 50 years that the number of cases becomes substantial. The incidence rises with age until in old age cerebrovascular accidents become a major cause of death.

A cerebrovascular accident, in the majority of cases, is abrupt in onset and marked signs may become evident in a matter of seconds or minutes. It is this very rapid onset which allows a highly probable inference of a vascular lesion. Occasionally the signs, slight at first, may steadily advance for a matter of hours, especially in the case of haemorrhage.

Of the clinical signs a loss of consciousness and a hemiplegia are much the most common. The term ' hemiplegia ' means a weakness of any degree of the face, arm and leg of one side. All the parts may be equally affected or one part may be more or less affected than others. As a rule there is some correspondence between the face and arm in their degree of weakness but the leg may be much stronger or weaker than the other parts. The reason for this is that the

---

* This is really a misnomer. Softening is a better term.

face and arm areas of the motor cortex are supplied by the middle cerebral artery while the leg area is supplied by the anterior cerebral artery.

The tendon jerks and muscle tone are variable in the early stages of a cerebrovascular accident. They may be either increased or diminished but within hours, days or weeks an increase is the rule.

Hemianaesthesia, hemianopia and the various neuropsychological signs, although less common than unconsciousness and hemiplegia, may be present. The association of signs is variable but some correlations are common.

1. If consciousness is lost, LT motor signs on one side or part of one side are nearly always evident. The reverse is not true for there may be a profound hemiplegia without the slightest impairment of consciousness.

2. When the weakness is found in the face and arm of the right side in a right-handed patient there is usually some degree of aphasia. Aphasia, however, may be present without weakness.

3. Inattention, dementia and amnesia as a rule do not appear as isolated signs but are discovered when a patient recovers from unconsciousness.

4. Hemianaesthesia (achoraesthesia) and hemianopia rarely appear as isolated signs.

It has been previously mentioned that a weakness of one side may follow a convulsion and it is perhaps obvious that from weakness developing rapidly in this way a cerebrovascular accident can be inferred with only a low probability. Nevertheless, it should be remembered that the first sign of a cerebrovascular accident may be a convulsion. The diagnosis in this event is bound to be difficult and will depend on the further evolution of signs, for with a neoplasm, for example, the signs will increase while with a vascular lesion they will diminish or remain static.

Occasionally a patient, without convulsions, complains of transient attacks of weakness of one side, or part of one side, lasting for minutes or hours. Such attacks were omitted from the classification of patients with seizures. It is advisable to speculate that all such attacks of weakness are due to ischaemia of a cerebral hemisphere and to investigate each case with this in mind.

The prediction of death or survival.—The reason for putting these predictions at the head of a list of inferences is that the neurosurgical investigations required to verify an intracerebral haematoma carry a certain risk. Should it be predicted that the patient will die then any investigation and treatment is justified but if survival is predicted then a certain degree of caution is called for.

Two pieces of evidence are important in the prediction of death and survival and these are level of unconsciousness 12 hours after onset and the degree of hemiplegia. A patient may rapidly sink into grades 1 and 2 of unconsciousness at the onset of a stroke but quickly rise to grades 3 and 4. The level of unconsciousness at the onset is not important. It is the level 12 hours after the onset that is important for patients who are in grades 1 and 2 at that time almost invariably die, while those who are in grade 4 almost invariably live. Patients who are in grade 3 have a roughly fifty-fifty chance of survival.

When patients are in grade 3 the severity of the hemiplegia assumes importance. Should a patient be partially paralysed in all parts of one side or completely paralysed in arm or leg, he has a four out of ten chance of survival but otherwise his chances are six out of ten. These probabilities unfortunately are not good enough for practical purposes.

Death, when it is predicted, nearly always occurs within two or three weeks.

The prognosis of ultimate disability.—It has already been said that the neurosurgical investigation (arteriography and needling of the brain) of a cerebrovascular accident are not without risk and these investigations cannot be justified if it can be predicted that the patient will make a satisfactory recovery. Unfortunately the prognosis of ultimate disability is much more difficult than that of death or survival. Hemiplegia, hemi-achoraesthesia, hemianopia, aphasia, dementia, agnosia and seizures may all constitute disabilities. Clearly it is asking a great deal to make a confident prognosis for each. At the moment we will attempt a prognosis for only a hemiplegia and aphasia.

A prognostic rule for cerebrovascular accidents is that the sooner some improvement becomes apparent the less the ultimate disability. Thus the return of even a little power within a few hours indicates that even a severe hemiplegia will ultimately disappear. On the other hand, the absence of even a slight return of power at the end of a week indicates that no recovery or only slight recovery will take place. In this assessment of future disability you should be on the look-out for a certain pitfall. Some patients, days after the onset of the stroke, appear to have a persistent severe paralysis of an arm inasmuch as they make little effort to use the arm even on examination. Nevertheless these patients, when they are coaxed to exert their greatest force in tests of strength, will be found to have almost normal strength. In the course of your examination you may in fact have the impression that the patient has forgotten how to use his arm or that, to put it colloquially, he cannot be bothered to use it. Uselessness of a hand is a fairly common permanent disability. This uselessness is often due to achoraesthesia and not to paralysis, a point worth remembering since, if the former is overlooked, the disability may be puzzling and much useless physiotherapy may be advised.

The prognosis for aphasia, to some degree, follows the same rule as that for hemiplegia. Nevertheless the degree of recovery is sometimes unexpected. Prognosis obviously depends, both for hemiplegia and aphasia, on the medical and nursing care which has been brought to bear, on the physiotherapy and speech therapy which has been instituted and last, but not least, on the intelligence and personality of the patient. The prognosis of ultimate disability has therefore to take several factors into account and much experience is required before a clinician can hope to become expert.

The differential diagnosis of infarct and haemorrhage.—A patient who dies within 24 hours of the onset of a stroke nearly always has had a haemorrhage but to make a diagnosis on the basis of death is to be wise after the event. Both an infarct and haemorrhage may present with dramatic suddenness or evolve slowly over some hours but it can be accepted that the latter evolution raises the probability of haemorrhage. Haemorrhage quickly causes a rise of intracranial pressure and may evoke headache and vomiting before consciousness is lost. Furthermore the pupils may enlarge as a result of coning. Leakage of blood into the subarachnoid space may produce neck stiffness and obviously, too, this blood may be demonstrated by lumbar puncture. Such signs, unfortunately, are absent in some cases of intracerebral haemorrhage.

Site of the lesion.—The site of the lesion is unimportant unless neurosurgery is contemplated. The great majority of patients have weakness on one side and consequently it is easy to infer which cerebral hemisphere is affected. Should the face and arm be very weak while the leg remains strong it can be inferred that the lesion is within the territory of the middle cerebral artery. On the other hand, weakness of the leg while the face and arm remain strong allows an inference of a lesion within the territory of the anterior cerebral artery. If all parts are equally weak the territory of both arteries must be affected although it must be remembered that a relatively small lesion in the internal capsule produces the same effect as a large lesion nearer the surface of the cerebrum.

An infarction in the territory of the posterior cerebral artery is unusual. It is associated with only a momentary slight impairment of consciousness and the only neurological sign is a homonymous hemianopia. This hemianopia is usually incomplete but unfortunately is generally permanent. The latter part of this statement is, however, based on the cases referred to hospital and may not be true of all cases.

With infarction the site of the blocked vessel is always proximal to the site of the infarcted brain. There are therefore two sites of lesions to be inferred, a neurological and a vascular. An infarction in the territory of the middle cerebral artery may be caused by a block in the middle cerebral artery itself, at its junction with the carotid artery, or by a block in the internal carotid artery at any part of its course although the point of origin of the internal and external carotid arteries is the most common. The more proximal the block the greater is the opportunity for collateral circulation to become effective although the effectiveness of this collateral circulation depends on anatomical variations, the health of the collateral arteries and the efficiency of the general circulation.

The site of a thrombosed vessel can rarely be diagnosed without the help of arteriography except in the case of the carotid artery. The origin of the internal and external carotid arteries is a common site of atheroma and as a result the circulation through the internal carotid artery may become gradually reduced. This may be compensated by collateral circulation but should this fail intermittently for one reason or another the patient may experience transient symptoms. These may be in the form of brief impairment of consciousness, of diminution of vision in the eye on the same side as the obstructed artery due to failure in the circulation through the ophthalmic artery, or transient weakness or achoraesthesia of the opposite limbs, especially the arm and more especially the hand.

When the blockage of the internal carotid artery becomes complete the clinical picture is variable depending again on the effectiveness of the collateral circulation. There may be no symptoms whatever or the patient may become deeply unconscious with a profound hemiplegia or there may be any clinical state between these two extremes. In short, the clinical picture is that of a cerebral infarction and from this picture a block of the internal carotid artery cannot be inferred with a high probability. It is only when signs are transient and relatively slight that the probability rises.

The apparent absence of pulsation of a carotid artery and the presence of bruits are not reliable signs of a complete or partial occlusion of the artery respectively. The arterial pressure of the retinal vessels is considered to be a better guide but this is outside the scope of the student.

Brain-stem vascular accidents.—You should refresh your memory of the brain-stem arteries and you should note that the posterior cerebral arteries are end-branches of the basilar artery. Complete or partial occlusion of the basilar artery produces anoxia of the anterior portions of the pons and as a result there may be unilateral or bilateral LT motor signs. With the former the ultimate prognosis is poor and with the latter the immediate prognosis is poor. With bilateral lesions dysarthria is often produced and this should not be confused with aphasia, a mistake liable to be made when the LT motor signs are much more marked on the right side. Permanent visual loss may also be present.

Blockage of the arteries supplying the posterior parts of the brain-stem rarely produce syndromes which allow the affected artery to be identified but an exception is a thrombosis of the posterior inferior cerebellar artery. This brain-stem lesion presents a good exercise

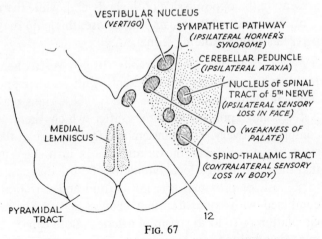

Fig. 67

The Territory of the Posterior Inferior Cerebellar Artery.

in neurological signs and, by referring to Figure 67 which shows the territory supplied by this artery, the clinical picture can be synthesised. The condition begins with acute vertigo which may last for hours or days. There is a loss of pain sense in the face on the same side as the affected artery and on the opposite side of the body. This so-called crossed anaesthesia allows a very high probability inference of a pontine lesion. There is often nystagmus, a weak palate and hoarseness of the voice (due to a 10th nerve lesion on the same side), a Horner's syndrome and a cerebellar ataxia on the same side as the affected artery. You should note that the pyramidal tracts and the medial lemniscus are un-affected and consequently the patient does not exhibit weakness or achoraesthesia. Lastly, it may be mentioned that diffuse disagreeable pain (thalamic pain) may be present on the opposite side of the body and, while there is often considerable recovery otherwise, this pain may persist as a long-standing sequel.

Transient anoxia of nervous tissue.—A frequent problem is a patient who presents with sudden and transient signs referable to the brain. These signs may last seconds, minutes or hours after which there is complete recovery. The transient and focal nature of the signs suggests a focal anoxia and this in turn suggests that there has been a local circulatory failure due either to stenosis of proximal arteries (carotid and vertebral) combined with some transient change in the general circulation or to local spasm of arteries. Both causes, it must be admitted, are speculative.

Transient weakness, paraesthesiae or achoraesthesia of limbs and face on one side, aphasia or agnosia would seem to be almost certainly due to focal cerebral anoxia. There are, however, numerous signs and combinations of signs which would seem to implicate the brain-stem arteries. Among these signs are vertigo, cerebellar ataxia, bilateral weakness (and dysarthria), diplopia, bilateral paraesthesiae and also, it should be noted, visual disorders. The last should occasion no surprise when the source of the posterior cerebral arteries is remembered. There is a great variety of visual disorders and these have been touched upon in relation to migraine. It follows that the elements of migraine, other than the headache, may often be explained by spasm of brain-stem arteries.

Paroxysmal disorders are often found in young adults, occasionally in children, and it seems unlikely that atheroma and transient general circulatory failure can be held to account for the majority of such cases. Arterial spasm, therefore, seems a more reasonable speculative cause for focal anoxia in young people. The cause of arterial spasm has, however, yet to be found and for the time being we may speculate that the immediate cause of spasm lies in the activity of the nervous supply of arteries while the remote cause may lie in the realm of mental states. The latter should not seem absurd, for people sometimes become pale with fear. This takes us to psychosomatic disorders which will be discussed later.

Aneurysms.—The majority of aneurysms occur in the region of the anterior part of the circle of Willis where they are in close relation with the 2nd, 3rd, 4th, 5th and 6th nerves. The symptoms may be sudden in onset and consist of pain either in the forehead or behind an eye and possibly diplopia. On examination weakness of the extrinsic eye muscles and ptosis may be found and in addition there may be a loss of sensation in the first division of the 5th nerve. When the evolution of signs is slow an aneurysm cannot be differentiated from any other tumour.

Aneurysms in the middle and anterior cerebral arteries produce no compressive effects.

When an aneurysm bursts, the blood spills into the subarachnoid space and occasionally it bursts its way into the cerebrum. In the case of the middle and anterior cerebral arteries the loss of circulation due to an aneurysm bursting in their course may add a cerebral infarction to the other types of lesions.

A subarachnoid haemorrhage may cause a sudden loss of consciousness although some patients have a preliminary period of headache and less commonly of vomiting. Indeed in some patients the headache and vomiting may be the only symptoms. On examination, apart from impairment of consciousness, the only other sign which is commonly found is neck stiffness. Blood in the CSF, of course, is the definition of a subarachnoid haemorrhage and when it is found the diagnosis is not a matter of inference. Occasionally the addition of intracerebral haemorrhage and infarction makes the clinical picture a less simple one and weakness, aphasia and so on may be found. The local compressive effects of an aneurysm on cranial nerves may also be present.

Subarachnoid haemorrhage carries a heavy mortality although it must be made clear that this statement, like all others so far made on cerebrovascular conditions, is based on hospital cases and as such represent the most severe forms of such conditions. As with cerebral infarction and haemorrhage, grades 1 and 2 of unconsciousness persisting over 12 hours substantially worsens the prognosis for life although, unlike the cerebral conditions, patients with subarachnoid haemorrhage occasionally survive. Focal cerebral signs, which no doubt indicate intracerebral haemorrhage or infarction, lower the probability of survival and to such adverse signs can be added hypertension and a rise of temperature.

Paralysis agitans

Paralysis agitans or Parkinsonism is a name for evidence from which a disorder of the basal ganglia may be inferred with a high probability. The patient's appearance in the late stages of the disease is very striking but in the early stages close scrutiny must be given to the signs about to be enumerated if the condition is not to be overlooked.

There is an immobility of facial muscles especially those around the eyes. Although the patient blinks fairly readily there is a curious fixity of the orbicularis oculi which becomes more evident if attention is given to the eyebrows which will be observed to move very little. Of course, there is no paralysis of the facial muscles and all parts can be moved fully when the patient endeavours to do so.

A patient with paralysis agitans remains quite still as you interview him. He does not fidget or alter his position or posture from time to time as people usually do as they are sitting. This general immobility is the most obtrusive sign and is sometimes referred to as a poverty of movement. As the patient stands it is noticeable, at least in a fairly advanced case, that the trunk and limbs assume a semi-flexed posture and this is maintained even on walking unless the patient chooses to alter it. This appearance is made more striking on walking for the patient shuffles his feet and at the same time fails to swing his arms.

There are other signs which deserve special mention.

Muscular rigidity.—On passive movement a resistance is experienced which is different from that found with LT motor lesions. With paralysis agitans the resistance, now called rigidity rather than spasticity, is maintained throughout the range of movement and is sometimes referred to as lead-pipe rigidity for this reason. In the arms two special techniques are useful in demonstrating this rigidity. The examiner clasps the patient's hand as in an ordinary handshake and with the patient's forearm maintained at 90° at the elbow the forearm is alternately pronated and supinated. This should be done at varying speeds since there is an optimum speed for each patient. In the second test the examiner clasps the patient's wrist with one hand and the patient's finger with the other hand. He then alternately extends and flexes the wrist, again at varying speeds. These tests may also reveal a cog-wheel rigidity which is due to a combination of rigidity and tremor, the latter being not necessarily visible.

Tremor.—The tremor of paralysis agitans is coarse and slow and as such is quite different from the tremor of hyperthyroidism. It varies a great deal in amplitude between patients and at different times in the same patient. It is present at rest but not during sleep and is minimised by voluntary movement unless such movements are made when the patient is nervous or embarrassed. The tremor in the hands sometimes assumes a pill-rolling appearance for the semi-flexed thumb is seen to pass over the tips of the semi-flexed fingers.

Dysarthria.—The speech may become slow and assume an unvarying pitch. Phonation may also become weak and the words poorly articulated.

Loss of dexterity of movement.—Clumsiness of movement may sometimes be found even in the absence of rigidity and tremor. This clumsiness is evident in all parts but tests should be confined to the hands and they should not be performed until tests of strength have been completed. The loss of dexterity may often constitute the greatest disability.

It should be noted that there is no causal correlation between poverty of movement, rigidity, tremor and clumsiness for one may be found without the others or in excess of others. The rigidity and tremor may occur only on one side or in one limb. It should also be remembered that in paralysis agitans there are no LT motor and sensory signs or cerebellar signs.

Patients themselves are rarely aware of the poverty of movement or of the semi-flexed posture. It is nearly always tremor or difficulty in walking that takes them to the doctor although they will often admit a general physical slowness. They may complain of cramp-like feelings in the muscles and if this is their only complaint the clinician may be misled. The evolution of the disease may be extremely slow over many years and the patient may reach an advanced stage without his relatives being aware that a physical disability has imposed itself. The patient indeed may be thought to be suffering from a psychiatric condition as he sits motionless, expressionless and huddled up at his fireside. His attitude admittedly is one of depression and even an admission of depression, a not unnatural mental state in view of the severity of the disability, should not excuse the clinician from performing a physical examination.

It has already been said that paralysis agitans is a name for evidence. Unfortunately clinicians will not adhere to a strict definition and the name is applied no matter what combination of signs is present. When clinicians abuse terms in this way it is often because they are thinking in terms of the inference and in the present case they are thinking of a disorder of the basal ganglia. The term thus comes to signify both the evidence and the inference and although this should be avoided it produces no great confusion with regard to paralysis agitans.

The pathology which causes paralysis agitans is still a matter of controversy but it is thought that the signs are produced by a functional disorder of the globus pallidus and that this is secondary to histological changes in the substantia nigra. Certainly histological changes in the basal ganglia of a neoplastic, infective or vascular type will not produce the syndrome and consequently the only pathological inference that can be made from the evidence is of a degenerative type. This simplifies the clinical diagnostic problem considerably. It may perhaps be repeated that the signs constituting paralysis agitans are nearly always found in isolation. Sometimes when the paralysis agitans is a sequel to an encephalitis other neurological signs may be found but these are rarely of a focal cerebral type.

CHAPTER XXX

DIFFUSE INTRACRANIAL LESIONS

Meningitis*

Several organisms are capable of causing meningitis but the meningococcus, *H. influenzae,* tubercle bacillus and several types of virus are the commonest pathogenic agents. Meningococcal and influenzal meningitis is still common in sporadic form whereas tuberculous meningitis is becoming relatively rare. Aseptic (or lymphocytic) meningitis, commonly due to a virus, sometimes occurs in small epidemics.

Meningococcal meningitis is an acute infection. The signs and symptoms evolve rapidly in a matter of hours and in a fulminating infection the patient may die of a septicaemia before neurological signs become evident. Tuberculous meningitis has a slower evolution over days while the onset of a viral meningitis, like the meningococcal type, is fairly abrupt.

The constitutional signs and symptoms of infection are present in most cases of meningitis and to this it is worth adding that apathy is often combined with irritability. This irritability or resentment of interference is not found in the intracranial diseases so far described, with the exception of intracerebral and subarachnoid

---

* Meningitis and encephalitis will be given in greater detail by your teacher of infectious diseases.

haemorrhage, in both of which it is an occasional finding.

Whatever the causal organism the superficial clinical picture of meningitis is fairly stereotyped. The patient, who feels miserably ill and distressed with headache, lies curled up on his side with the strong wish, it would seem, to be left alone. If the condition is allowed to progress, apathy may give way to loss of consciousness. Cerebral segmental signs apart from inattention, unconsciousness and possibly convulsions are minimal. Focal cerebral signs too are very unusual and when they do occur they are generally attributed to a concomitant cerebral infarction. It is the absence of focal signs which allows a distinction to be made between meningitis and cerebral abscess.

There is one sign of meningitis which is almost invariable and this is neck stiffness. To demonstrate neck stiffness, especially in its milder degrees, requires practice and your teacher will describe a suitable technique. This neck stiffness is also found to a marked degree in subarachnoid haemorrhage and is therefore not diagnostic of an infective meningitis. A sign, after all, indicates the site of a lesion and not its type. Neck stiffness too may be found with a cerebral abscess although here it may be argued that there is an element of meningitis. Any painful condition of the back of the head or neck, whether produced by an organic lesion or not, may be associated with neck stiffness but, when the pain is recent, subarachnoid haemorrhage and meningitis should always be considered. Lastly, neck stiffness may be found in the toxaemic states associated with pneumonia and in this case is referred to as meningismus. You will thus see that neck stiffness considered as an isolated sign does not have much significance but combined with the constitutional signs of infection it raises the probability of meningitis greatly. The absence of neck stiffness on the other hand, unless the patient is moribund, lowers the probability of meningitis almost to zero.

The CSF should always be examined when there is even a faint suspicion of meningitis. The findings have a profound effect on the probability of inference of meningitis and, apart from this, the causal organism may be either demonstrated or inferred from the nature of the CSF abnormalities. The CSF will be discussed later.

Meningococcal and tuberculous meningitis should be diagnosed at an early stage and treatment instituted. You will therefore not have the opportunity of observing the natural evolution of these diseases but this no doubt will be described in your course of instruction on infectious diseases. Even when infection is eradicated with antibiotics, however, there is a development which is worth mentioning since its occasional occurrence complicates the picture of meningitis. This is the production of adhesions at the base of the brain. These adhesions block the flow of CSF and cause a pressure hydrocephalus with its attendant signs. Indeed, the permanent sequelae of meningitis such as dementia and blindness often have meningeal adhesions as their immediate cause although, of course, the inflammation of the meninges is the remote cause.

Encephalitis

Encephalitis is a fairly diffuse inflammatory condition of the cerebrum and brain-stem. It is probably always due to a virus although the presence of such an organism can rarely be verified. It may rarely occur in epidemics (encephalitis lethargica) or as a complication of such diseases as measles and mumps and in these circumstances the diagnosis is readily apparent. Sometimes, however, it occurs sporadically and it is then that the diagnosis may be elusive. The acute phase of the disease usually runs a course of a few weeks or months, if death does not supervene, but months or years later certain sequelae may become evident.

Encephalitis is generally an acute infection, the signs and symptoms developing over a few hours or days. The constitutional signs and symptoms of infection may introduce or accompany the neurological signs or may be absent altogether.

The presenting picture of encephalitis varies a good deal. Thus, the first evidence of the disease may be fluctuations in the level of consciousness, behaviour and personality changes, convulsions or the constitutional signs of infection coupled with delirium. In the early stages, therefore, especially with sporadic cases, the disease may mislead even the best diagnostician.

In the fully developed case the signs are mostly of a cerebral segmental type. The patient may exhibit inattention, unconsciousness, dementia, amnesia and to this list may be added psychotic features such as disturbed behaviour and hallucinations. A common feature, unless the patient is deeply unconscious, is restlessness or delirium and this, it is worth noting, is unusual with neoplasms, vascular accidents and cerebral abscesses. Associated with the delirium may be a reversal of the sleep rhythm. Focal cerebral signs such as hemiplegia and aphasia are unusual but involuntary movements are fairly common.

The clinical picture, it will be seen, is not stereotyped. As a rule, CSF changes are sufficient to distinguish encephalitis from all other cerebral diseases which develop rapidly, with the exception of cerebral abscess, and to draw a distinction between the two conditions the clinician may have to resort to neuro-radiology and needling of the brain.

There are many sequelae to encephalitis. The most common is paralysis agitans and this may be associated with oculogyric crises in which the eyes deviate involuntarily for some minutes. Choreic and athetotic movements may persist and in other patients tics or habit spasms may make their appearance. Other sequelae are major convulsive seizures, psychical seizures, dementia and asocial behaviour.

Subacute encephalitis is a type of encephalitis which deserves special mention. This disease occurs in children usually between the ages of 5 and 15 years and proceeds to death in about two years. It usually presents with dementia and the features of a psychosis but within a few months myoclonus makes its appearance and this may be associated with petit mal. The patient steadily deteriorates and eventually becomes moribund. This is the only organic cerebral disease in which the EEG raises the probability of the inference almost to certainty.

General paralysis of the insane

General paralysis of the insane (G.P.I.) is a diffuse cerebral disease of adults caused by the *Treponema pallidum* and makes its appearance years after the primary infection. It evolves slowly over months and years and there is a progressive deterioration unless the natural evolution is interrupted by treatment.

The constitutional signs of infection are absent. In the early stages the evidence consists only of psychological disturbances which are apparent only to the patient's close associates. Such disturbances are described in terms of mental slowness, failure of judgment and so on. You should refer to the lay terminology given in Figure 56. By the time the patient comes under medical care dementia and amnesia have become apparent. In due course all types of cerebral segmental signs may make their appearance and eventually LT motor signs may be superimposed.

G.P.I. has become relatively uncommon and few clinicians have seen a sufficient number of cases to become expert in diagnosis. Fortunately other evidence of neurosyphilis may accompany the signs of G.P.I. and this will often assist the clinician in reaching the correct diagnosis. Thus the patient may have Argyll Robertson pupils, optic atrophy or loss of tendon jerks. Indeed, the signs of tabes dorsalis may be quite marked and their association with G.P.I. justifies the term tabo-

171

paresis. Even when signs are minimal, however, the probability of G.P.I. can be substantially raised or lowered by the WR which is positive in blood or CSF in all cases. There may also be an increase of cells and protein in the CSF.

Pre-senile dementia

The term pre-senile dementia signifies a dementia occurring in middle age (40-60 years). The term covers a group of disorders which include Pick's disease, Alzheimer's disease and Jacob-Creutzfeldt's disease but the distinction between them is a matter for the expert and we will content ourselves with the common features. The underlying pathology is a diffuse or patchy atrophy of the cerebrum.

The condition is insidious in onset and slowly progresses to death over a course of several years. The earliest sign may be amnesia or dementia but before long both are present. The clinical picture can be given in terms of the lay terminology given in Figure 56. Any combination of cerebral segmental signs may be found, unconsciousness, however, occurring only in the terminal phases. Aphasia may be prominent and also dysarthria. The latter is explained by bilateral lesions in the cerebral motor pathways which may also produce a pseudo-bulbar palsy.

As the disease progresses the patient's movements may become slower and this, with a loss of facial expression and rigidity of muscles, results in a state reminiscent of paralysis agitans although the association of dementia is sufficient to exclude the latter condition.

Cerebral arteriosclerosis

Apart from infarction and haemorrhage the brain may show widespread slow degeneration as a result of arteriosclerosis. The patient may therefore present with a slowly progressive dementia and amnesia. Other neuro-psychological signs and LT signs may slowly emerge or develop abruptly as a result of infarction. Psychological signs, too, may be superimposed. Occasionally Parkinsonism complicates the picture.

The distinction between this condition and pre-senile dementia rests largely on other evidence of cardiovascular disease and also on the occasional abrupt aggravation of symptoms and signs which are the product of small infarctions.

Huntington's chorea

This is an inherited disease which usually first becomes evident between the ages of 30 and 50 years. The disease presents a mixture of dementia and chorea although some members of a family may show only one feature or, in a particular member, one feature may precede the other.

The chorea, at first slight, affects mainly the face, shoulders and arms. As it progresses, the jerking movements increase in amplitude and interfere with voluntary movements. Facial expressions may be obscured while speech may assume a choreic jerkiness in both rhythm and pitch.

173

Cerebral segmental signs consist chiefly of dementia and amnesia, the former being more advanced than the latter. Inattention may be marked. Superimposed on these features or even preceding them there may be disorders of thought and emotion leading sometimes to violent behaviour or suicide.

Schilder's disease (diffuse sclerosis)

Schilder's disease is a rare condition which can occur at any age although the majority of cases begin before the age of 25 years. It consists of a diffuse demyelination of the cerebrum and possibly of the cerebellum. The demyelination usually begins anteriorly or posteriorly in the cerebrum, although as a rule fairly symmetrically, so that there is some variation in the presenting signs. The rate of progress, too, is variable, some cases advancing rapidly to death in a matter of months while others may progress slowly over years.

When the demyelination begins posteriorly the first evidence of the disease is hemianopic visual defects which may be unilateral in the early stages but become bilateral as the condition advances. When the demyelination begins anteriorly LT motor signs, eventually bilateral, develop and dysarthria may be prominent. Whatever the mode of onset cerebral segmental signs are not long delayed and eventually dominate the picture. It is worth noting that some cases show a slight swelling of the optic disks and in others cerebellar signs may be present, features which complicate the diagnostic problem.

174

Wilson's disease (Progressive lenticular degeneration)

Wilson's disease is a rare condition sometimes occurring in several members of one family. The disease, which begins in adolescence or childhood, runs a variable course and occasionally progresses to death in a few months but usually in a matter of years.

The clinical picture superficially resembles a paralysis agitans with the important difference that tremor is prominent and almost invariable. The tremor, too, may be complicated by choreo-athetoid movements and furthermore is aggravated, and not relieved, by voluntary movements. The rigidity is less constant than that of paralysis agitans for a superimposed athetosis gives the impression that the rigidity fluctuates. The rigidity is associated with slowness of movement and with postural distortions (flexion of arms and extension of legs). There is a fixity of expression round the eyes and this with a frequent smile gives the face an appearance described as a silly vacuous look. The speech becomes progressively dysarthric and this may be associated with a pseudo-bulbar palsy.

Some degree of dementia is generally found, although it is said to be rarely severe, and, if with this the patient is emotionally facile, the general behaviour may be described as childish.

There are two important diagnostic points which must be mentioned. Some patients show a brownish pigmentation at the edge of the cornea (the Kayser-Fleischer ring) and this is pathognomonic of the disease. The second point is that patients with the disease show an excessive excretion of copper in the urine, figures over 200 μg. per day being usual (normal 60 μg.).

Wernicke's encephalopathy

This condition, which is due to a deficiency of thiamin, may be secondary to malnutrition, alcoholism or gastric carcinoma. When mild, the condition is easily overlooked for depression or irritability may be thought to be the result of physical weakness. However, the appearance of dementia and amnesia make an organic cerebral condition highly probable although, of course, something more is required before Wernicke's encephalopathy can be considered. Nystagmus is said to be almost invariable while various combinations of 3rd, 4th and 6th nerve palsies are common. A polyneuritis too may be present. This rather strange combination of dementia, eye signs and polyneuritis makes a Wernicke's encephalopathy highly probable and even this probability is raised if some causal condition, such as those enumerated above, can be identified.

Hepatic encephalopathy

With acute hepatic failure, whatever the cause, the patient in the terminal stages becomes demented and consciousness is impaired. This gives rise to a picture often described as one of confusion, disorientation and delirium. Associated with this state there may be an increase of tendon jerks and a rather characteristic (but not pathognomonic) tremor, often referred to as a flapping tremor. This is produced when the patient stretches out his hands. Impairment of consciousness progresses until grade 1 is reached when death is not far off. Should the failure of the liver progress over weeks or months the evolution of neurological signs will be correspondingly slower. Apathy and confusion may last for several weeks before unconsciousness supervenes.

With acute and subacute failure of the liver the neurological signs rarely lead to diagnostic difficulty since there is usually abundant evidence of liver disease. Diagnostic difficulties only emerge when a patient with liver cirrhosis, and especially one who has had a portal caval shunt, lives on the point of liver failure, for marked neurological signs may develop without obvious evidence of advance in the liver disease. In such a patient neurological signs may be precipitated by the ingestion of large amounts of meat, by gastric haemorrhage and by the taking of hypnotics. The patient may rapidly become unconscious but fortunately this causes the ingestion of protein to be temporarily interrupted so that, in a sense, the condition is self-curative. Sometimes, rather than becoming unconscious, the patient becomes confused and disorientated and whether this lasts for only a short period or for weeks or months the diagnosis may remain unconsidered if concomitant liver disease is not appreciated by the clinician. Occasionally an agnosia is more evident than dementia so that the appropriate tests should not be neglected. With the milder degrees of a hepatic encephalopathy the patient may exhibit only minor personality changes but such changes are usually no

177

THE INFERENCE OF CEREBRAL PATHOLOGY FROM CLINICAL EVIDENCE

Disease	Pathology		Age	Evolution	Non-neurological	Signs				CSF
	Focal	Diffuse				LT	Neuro-psychological (include seizures)	Psychological		
Neoplasm										
Abscess										
Vascular accident										
Meningitis										
Encephalitis										
G.P.I.										
Pre-senile dementia										
Cerebral arteriosclerosis										
Huntington's chorea										
Schilder's disease										
Wilson's disease										
Wernicke's encephalopathy										
Hepatic encephalopathy										

Fig. 68

more than a prelude to the more serious disturbances already described. The characteristic feature of this encephalopathy is the fluctuation in the severity of the signs, sometimes from hour to hour. This, of course, is not diagnostic since it may occur in any intoxication but it should obviously arouse the suspicions of the clinician when no cause of intoxication is apparent.

Conclusion

Although Chapters XXIX and XXX contain descriptions of many diseases there are yet others which you should be familiar with. These can be put under the headings of toxic and metabolic cerebral disorders and are more suitably described by general physicians.

In your first reading of Chapters XXIX and XXX you will probably find it difficult to memorise the important and common features of each disease. A useful exercise is to complete Figure 68.

CHAPTER XXXI

PSYCHOSOMATIC DISORDERS

Emotional states as causes of somatic disorders

Previously we have been working on the assumption that all somatic disorders have physical causes. We have now to turn our attention to a group of disorders, exemplified by headache and indigestion, which many clinicians believe have mental causes. There is no general agreement about the definition of psychosomatic disorder but the following one will allow us to make a start on this difficult and important aspect of clinical medicine.

> A psychosomatic disorder is a bodily feeling (*e.g.* indigestion) or bodily state (*e.g.* peptic ulcer) which is caused by mental states or, more precisely, by unpleasant emotional states.

You will notice that the definition contains an effect and its cause but we will let this pass since we have enough difficulties on hand.

Since we have so far progressed in an apparently satisfactory way you may possibly doubt the necessity of introducing mental causes. Admittedly many causal chains are satisfactory. Here is an example.

Organisms $\longrightarrow$ abscess $\longrightarrow$ swelling $\longrightarrow$ pain. But some chains, such as the following, seem incomplete.

? $\longrightarrow$ peptic ulcer $\longrightarrow$ indigestion.

This causal chain is incomplete in several respects. The cause of peptic ulcer is unknown; peptic ulcer alone is inadequate to explain indigestion, for people with continuous peptic ulcer have indigestion only intermittently; and, lastly, some people with indigestion have no peptic ulcer as far as can be ascertained. These points allow us to formulate three general problems, namely, the problems of the cause of bodily states and feelings when no causal bodily states or environmental conditions are known and the problem of the cause of bodily feelings when known causal bodily states do not constitute complete explanations.

In trying to solve these problems we may, of course, continue to search exclusively for physical causes but, if this approach proves unprofitable, we may justifiably turn our attention to mental states and try to discover whether or not they form links in causal chains. It may be remarked at this point that, although there appears to be a clear distinction between physical and mental states, the nature of this distinction on closer inquiry is somewhat elusive.

Previously it has been stated that a patient's saying that he has a pain, for example, and his behaving as if he had a pain can be used as evidence from which inferences may be drawn. But at the moment we are trying to establish mental states as causes and it is clear that in this endeavour the substitution of *saying that* and *behaving as if* evidence for the mental states themselves can only be allowed with certain reservations. It may, indeed, seem to you that since other peoples' mental states cannot be observed and, since it is inconceivable that they ever will be, the study of mental states is outwith the limits of empirical science. We may, nevertheless, try to keep the study of mental states within these limits by a process of analogical thinking. Consider the following proposition.

I have observed (I am aware) on one occasion that a man (myself) who laughs $\xrightarrow{\quad 1 \quad}{1}$ is feeling happy.*

Can I now infer that, when you laugh, you are feeling happy? The answer to this question is based on the empirical rule that the stronger the analogy between the objects of a correlative proposition the more reliable the inferences or, more accurately, the more reliable the probabilities. To put the matter in another way, the stronger the analogy the fewer the number of objects necessary in a correlative proposition for

---

* We may translate this proposition into one in which the numerical probability refers to the number of observations and not to the number of objects observed.

I have observed (I am aware) on 100 occasions that a man (myself) who laughs $\xrightarrow{\quad 99 \quad}{100}$ is feeling happy.

By using this kind of proposition a cause in an individual object can be established. This obliges us to distinguish between individual and general causes. We must also enlarge our definition of property as follows.

A property is a point of similarity and difference between objects and between an object observed at different times.

reliable probabilities. With regard to our present example the analogy between people is very strong and consequently I may conclude that, when you laugh you are feeling happy. Of course, it may be objected that a reliable probability can hardly be derived from observations of one object and against this no defence can be sustained. Nevertheless, if we are to make any progress we must assume that the probability has a fair degree of reliability. For the sake of completeness it may be said that, when you say you are feeling happy, I am led to believe that you have a feeling similar to that when you laugh and, as already indicated, by analogical thinking I appreciate what your feelings are. To sum up therefore we may say that, although other people's mental states are not observable, we nevertheless know what these feelings are.

Lastly, on the basis that people are honest most of the time, we may conclude that inferences of mental states from statements and behaviour have a high probability. Now when an inference is almost certain it can be substituted, in any proposition, for the evidence from which it is derived without much error being introduced into the probability. Consequently the property of feeling happy, for example, can be used as evidence by substituting it for *saying that* and *behaving as if* evidence.

Having, to some degree, convinced ourselves that, contrary to first impressions, mental states can be used as evidence, we have now to establish them as causes. A moment's reflection reveals that, when we will a movement, the movement takes place; when we imagine an appetising meal our mouths water; and when we recall an embarrassing incident we blush. We therefore feel justified in saying that mental states are causes of bodily states. Our spontaneous conviction in the matter rests on the fact that the bodily state follows the mental state with such rapidity that no other property appears to be involved. But further consideration makes it plain that, despite the rapidity of the bodily response, the nervous system constitutes a large series of causal links between the mental state and its ultimate effect. Our conviction on speed of response being somewhat shaken, we are led to suspect that mental states themselves may be no more than side-effects of the nervous system. Observations on patients with cerebral lesions seem sufficient to establish the cerebrum as a cause of mental states but it is inconceivable what sort of observations would establish mental states as causes of cerebral states. In these circumstances the only reasonable speculation open to us is that cerebral states cause all mental states and that the latter are always effects and never causes. This can be shown diagrammatically.

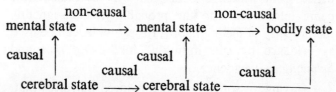

If, by adopting this speculation, we do not feel entitled to call mental states causes we can avoid the obvious difficulty of communication by using terms signifying mental states as symbols of the cerebral states which we suppose must cause them. Thus, when we say that anxiety causes indigestion we really mean that there is a cerebral state which causes both anxiety and indigestion. This is not so absurd as it first appears for a psychiatrist referring to the unconscious mind, an expression which seems to involve a contradiction, is probably referring to a cerebral state thus:

cerebral state ⟶ cerebral state ⟶ mental state
(unconscious mind)

We must stop now and consider how we would go about establishing a particular mental state as a cause of a particular somatic disorder. Let us take, as an example, anxiety as a cause of headache. No matter how well we design our experiment we are constantly faced with an insurmountable difficulty. The clinician's knowledge of a patient's mental states is derived largely from statements of the latter. But the sort of statements a patient makes depends on his intelligence, introspection and his ability to use words; and last, but not least, it depends on the kind of questions put to him. Terms signifying mental states are therefore rather vague. Now the reliability of probabilities in propositions depends a great deal on the precision of terms and an example will convince you of this. The probability contained in the statement that people with cerebrovascular accidents are nearly always old is unreliable since the term old is vague. The probability is shown to be unreliable when old is taken to mean any age over 90 years. It follows, therefore, that, if the probabilities of correlative propositions are unreliable, then pairs of propositions formulated to establish causes are invalid since the changes in probabilities are worthless statistically. Anxiety and headache, too, are very common symptoms and we would have to design our experiment so that the degree of these symptoms was taken into account. But, as already indicated, measurement of anxiety and headache is out of the question and so most experiments fail before they even start.

The only feasible method of establishing anxiety as a cause of headache is to divide a number of suitable subjects into two groups and then, by some means or other, remove the anxiety of one group. This would possibly give us the following propositions.

$$\text{People} \left\{ \begin{array}{l} \text{with anxiety and headache} \xrightarrow{\frac{80}{100}} \text{continue to have headache.} \\ \\ \text{with headache and who have anxiety removed} \xrightarrow{\frac{40}{100}} \text{continue to have headache.} \end{array} \right.$$

Anxiety is thereby established as a cause of headache. Of course, the experiment is open to many criticisms, some of which have already been indicated. A further important criticism, however, would be that perhaps some property other than anxiety has been removed during the course of the experiment and this certainly seems possible should there be a long interval between the removal of the anxiety and the cessation of the headache.

As a rule, in clinical practice, the search for unpleasant emotional states is pursued indirectly by searching for environmental conditions which the clinician thinks likely to provoke unpleasant emotions. When such conditions have been discovered the clinician then tries to discover the emotional reactions of the patient. Such an inquiry is valid although it carries with it the danger that the clinician is apt to project himself into the revealed environmental conditions and, should he suppose that such conditions would evoke unpleasant emotions in himself, he further supposes that they must also do so in the patient. This is clearly a *non sequitur*. It is perhaps needless to add that the association in time of environmental conditions, unpleasant emotions and somatic disorders does not show that the first two are causal links with the last as an effect. If there is any criticism we would wish to make of the psychiatrist's approach to psychosomatic disorders it would rest on this.

The search for uncongenial environmental conditions is a valid method in clinical medicine and no criticisms need necessarily be levelled at correlations between environmental conditions and somatic disorders. Criticisms, however, can be made when the clinician interposes a causal link in terms of mental states which the patient denies. This is a common practice among psychiatrists and their defence that such mental states may be unconscious is breached by the claim that unconscious mental states are generally speculative and that there is no conceivable way of verifying them.

There is a very large literature on psychosomatic disorders written for the most part by psychiatrists. You are well advised to be critical of everything you read although, of course, this should not diminish your sympathy for psychiatrists in their endeavours in a difficult and complex field. At the same time you need not feel obliged to accept the numerous pseudo-properties or, more correctly, pseudo-words which are introduced. Examples are tension, stress and strain and, like so many other words used in psychology, they refer to some analogy which is never clearly specified. Analogies, you should note, give us a sense of familiarity with a subject and a sense of familiarity gives us a feeling of understanding. But a feeling of understanding is delusive if weak analogy is its only foundation.

Rest-lessness as a cause of somatic disorders

Should we look for a common feature among people with headache we would find that they are nearly all busy people and, if we consider the term ' busy ' in this connection, we find that it means to be constantly occupied. It is perhaps obvious that a person may be occupied mentally or physically but the state which is common to both is one of alertness.

The state of alertness is an interesting one. It probably reaches its highest levels in competitive activities although in such circumstances it is generally called excitement or tension. To act, mentally or physically, at high speed seems to necessitate a high degree of alertness, the more automatic actions requiring less alertness than those still being learned. It is probably more accurate to say that it is speed of reaction rather than speed of action which is a necessary associate of high level alertness, for in a position of being the hunter or being hunted the physical state, and the mental state for that matter, may at times be one of immobility.

While it may be admitted that high level alertness is implied by fast reaction, it is also true that a high level of alertness is present when fast reaction would seem irrelevant to the situation. For example, a task which is being performed with care to avoid error demands a high level of alertness and this holds for both physical and mental acts for, as far as alertness is concerned, there is little difference between performing a surgical operation and playing a game of chess. Further to this argument it may be added that to watch or listen carefully, even when no reaction is contemplated, also demands a high level of alertness.

So far we have used the term alertness without offering a definition. Introspection reveals that alertness is sometimes associated with fear, anger or pleasure but often it has no emotional overtones and therefore cannot itself be identified as an emotional state. Further introspection reveals that alertness is no more than attentiveness, the two terms being synonymous. In other words, to be alert is to be attentive, and to be attentive is to direct or focus the attention on mental operations or external events. Perhaps at this point a definition of attentiveness is required but since this forms much the same problem as the definition of pain, for example, we will let the matter rest.

It is apparent from self-observation that alertness fluctuates a great deal during the waking hours. Its peak is no doubt reached in positions of mortal danger while the opposite state, that is to say the lowest level of alertness, occurs in rest. Indeed, we may take rest and the lowest level of alertness to be synonymous. Rest, in the sense we are now using the word, means a state of physical and mental passivity during which the attention is not focused or directed. In such a state the subject sees rather than observes and thoughts which pass through his mind may be described as idle or spontaneous since he is passive to them rather than directing them. This state of rest may be described as daydreaming but, as such, is not necessarily concerned with wishful-thinking. As a digression it may be said that this state of rest, with the eyes open, allows *alpha* waves in the EEG to emerge.

All organs in a sense may be said to work and this work is directed towards an end. With all organs, except the nervous system, the end may be analysed in mechanical and chemical terms. As examples, the kidneys excrete urine and the lungs oxygenate the blood. The end point of nervous work, however, is difficult to analyse and consequently it is difficult to assess the amount of work done by the nervous system. For present purposes the degree of alertness or attention may be taken as a measure of this work. On the basis of what has already been said it may now be stated that, the greater the speed and the more care, the higher is the level of alertness and consequently the greater is the degree of nervous work. Also, over a period of time the more sustained the alertness the more work is performed by the nervous system. In a nutshell, speed, care and continuity tax the nervous system and it may be speculated that beyond a certain point the nervous system cannot cope. To disagree with this is to aver that the nervous system has no limits and no breaking point.

When you talk to patients about their work you should attempt an analysis in terms of speed, care and continuity and not pay a great deal of attention to the amount of muscular work involved. Advice to patients about avoiding nervous fatigue should be based on the following rules.

1. A man performing a job at high speed must be allowed to make mistakes.

2. A man performing a job with much care must be allowed to take his time.

3. A man performing a job which requires high speed and much care must be allowed frequent rest periods.

Patients with psychosomatic complaints generally claim that they never feel tired or at least never sufficiently tired to bring physical and mental activity to a halt. You must make it clear to patients, therefore, that you are talking about fatigue of the nervous system (and especially of the brain) and not about a feeling.

191

It has been said that people with headaches are constantly occupied. We may therefore refer to them as rest-less people, hyphenating the word to distinguish it from *restless* which, by common usage, has a somewhat different meaning from that at present intended. You can readily confirm that people with headache are rest-less although in your interviews you should watch out for certain pitfalls. Patients with headache will often claim that they frequently rest, especially in the evenings, but when you inquire further you will find that during their periods of so-called rest, they are watching television, reading, talking, knitting, thinking in an active sort of way or performing some other activity. Sometimes, too, patients say that they rest when they mean that they sleep in a chair and in this connection it is worth remarking that the people we are at present considering readily fall asleep should they abandon their activities for a few minutes. This suggests that they alternate between two states, namely sleep and a fairly high level alertness.

Patients often use the words 'rest' and 'relaxation' as synonyms and this you will find introduces considerable confusion into your discussions when you realise that, to most patients, relaxation is an activity associated with pleasant emotions. If you insist on our present definition of rest, your patients with headache will be forced to admit that they never rest. They may in fact be incredulous that anyone can or would want to rest and they will probably defend their position by claiming that time is valuable and that it is a sin to waste time. And to these clichés they will no doubt add that you should never put off till tomorrow things which can be done today.

A clinician, living in a middle class society of European origin and spending his working day among patients suffering largely from psychosomatic disorders, would probably claim that all people are rest-less. This claim could be disputed on the ground that observations were not made on a random selection of the world's population but this argument will not be pursued. That rest-lessness has a causal relationship with headache would seem to be established by the well-known fact that people with headache and indigestion often obtain at least temporary relief from hospital rest. It could of course be argued that hospital admission removes more than rest-lessness and consequently the claim that rest-lessness causes headache is invalid. But until the other properties which are said to be removed are specified and verified this criticism must be judged not very strong.

Rest-lessness implies continuous moderate or high levels of alertness and this being so it is not unexpected that rest-less people are often meticulous, conscientious and hard-working. Psychiatrists would say that they are obsessional and perfectionists and to this the patients would reply that, if a thing is worth doing, it is worth doing well. You must realise, however, that not all rest-less people have the excellent qualities enumerated above for some are so easily distracted and restless that they are virtually unemployable, and there

193

are others who find it more convenient to expend their energy on anti-social and destructive acts. Some people, too, dissipate their energy in a multitude of trivial activities.

Should we quantify alertness, taking into account the levels of alertness and duration, then observations on people give the impression that each person's weekly or monthly quantity does not vary a great deal. During any particular week or month the quantity may of course fluctuate but the total quantity for each period varies little about the average for the individual. Some people, the so-called energetic ones, obviously maintain a greater quantity than others and this quantity appears to be an inherited feature. In other words, if we can imagine a neurological activity-stat which regulates the weekly or monthly quantity of alertness, we may suppose that this regulating device is set at birth. Thereafter, the environment, in the ordinary course of events, raises or lowers the setting only a little. And to this it must be added that, in terms of quantity of activity, people choose or make their own environments. We may now speculate that, when over a fairly long period of time, the quantity of alertness (or activity) exceeds the setting of the activity-stat, unpleasant somatic effects ensue. Observations to a slight degree verify this speculation for the onset or exacerbation of certain somatic disorders often coincides with periods of increased activity. Sometimes, too, patients recollect that, during the period prior to the onset or exacerbation of a somatic disorder, the level of activity which they have maintained for years seemed to call for greater effort and that they had ceased, as it were, to take things in their stride. Here we could perhaps speculate that advancing years, depression or concurrent illness had reduced the setting on the activity-stat so that it fell below the level of activity.

It is obvious that, in using the term ' activity-stat ', we are referring to a rather weak analogy and we should therefore not be too impressed with any feeling of understanding which the analogy may evoke. Clearly, to establish increased activity as a cause of headache it would be necessary to design an investigation which would allow a pair of propositions to be formulated. Such an investigation is extremely difficult to design and for the time being our speculations must remain substantially unverified.

Increased activity may be associated with pleasant or unpleasant emotions and it is in the case of the latter that there is the temptation to suppose that it is the emotion rather than the activity which is the causal property. You will find, when you make your own observations, that happy people are as prone to psychosomatic disorders as unhappy people and, apropos of previous remarks, you will find that bad people are as prone as good people; that successful people are as prone as unsuccessful people; and that stupid people are as prone as intelligent people.

Conclusion

We have discussed two speculative causes of certain somatic disorders. There is no necessary incompatibility between these speculations for it may be that unpleasant emotions are associated with or even cause rest-lessness or increased levels of alertness. The advantage of the speculation of rest-lessness and continuous high level alertness as causes is that it offers explanations when speculations of unpleasant emotions fail to satisfy.* In therapy, however, you can use either or both speculations as the occasion demands. Uncongenial environmental conditions and unpleasant emotions, like bad teeth, may do no harm but they are unlikely to do any good and it needs little justification to attempt their removal. If such attempts are ineffective, and they often are, then some attempt may be made to alter alertness. You will find that, attached as they are to the cliché that everything, which is worth doing, is worth doing well, most patients are unwilling or unable to reduce their level of alertness during physical or mental activity. For example, most typists find it distressing to type at less than their maximum speed. All that you can advise with any hope of success is that patients should introduce rest periods into their average day outside of working hours. You may further suggest that a man who works 10 to 12 hours a day has little time for hobbies, recreations and social activities and that only a small portion of his leisure time should be devoted to such pastimes. It may also be suggested that the 24 hours of each day should be divided between sleep, work, recreation and *rest* and that the division should be suitably adjusted for each

---

* Rest-lessness and high level alertness, unlike emotions, are also readily inferred from a person's behaviour.

individual. A weekly day of rest, too, can be recommended on the highest possible authority although our definition of rest may be a little too stringent.*

If this advice is rejected you can emphasise your point by declaring that alertness is the work or a measure of the work done by the nervous system, and pain, due to a functional disorder of the nervous system, is produced by a device built into the nervous system by means of which the subject is warned that his alertness, for too long a period, has been excessive. It may also be added that functional pain is a safety device which obliges the subject to rest or lower his level of alertness in order that his nervous system may be protected from overloading. It is easy, you will see, to invent weak analogies which convince the most stubborn. In employing these weak analogies, however, your conscience need not be troubled for your attempt to impose rest on a patient has the support of traditional medicine and orthodox practice.

Something must now be said about the identification of a condition as a psychosomatic disorder. To start with, it may be said that the term ' psychosomatic ' is a bad one, for combining, as it does, an effect and its cause, it gives the impression that certain bodily feelings and states are always caused by mental states. The truth is that certain feelings and states may sometimes be caused by mental states and sometimes not. For example, headache may sometimes be due to anxiety and sometimes to meningitis. The claim that

* Religious worship, at least in part, implies a state of passivity.

197

a certain kind of headache is due to anxiety and another due to meningitis is not only wrong but dangerous. Of course there may be one kind of headache which gives a highly probable inference of anxiety and another of meningitis but that is another matter and neither should be claimed as a cause until they are discovered in the individual patient. In practice a bodily feeling or state should be considered to have a physical cause until reasonable investigation has proved the contrary and it is only then that a search should be made for mental causes. It must be admitted that an investigation which is to be considered reasonable will vary with each type of case but this does not modify the meaning of the previous statement.

There is a strong temptation to speculate about mental states as links when the causal chains of certain conditions seem inadequate. To give way to this temptation should not be too strongly criticised provided, as indicated above, a reasonable attempt has been made to complete the chains with physical causes. In neurology there is certainly the temptation to look for mental causes in most cases of headache, paroxysmal vertigo, major non-convulsive seizures and in many other examples of paroxysmal and episodic disorders. Disseminated sclerosis may be included among the last but this will not be enlarged upon in case it should offend commonsense. As a rule it does not require much effort to discover that patients with these complaints are rest-less (and usually physically restless) and that increased activity precipitates or aggravates the symptoms. If the above remarks upset you it should be remembered, with regard to our present speculations, that mental states, at the most, are co-existent causes of certain somatic disorders and that to postulate mental causes is not to deny physical causes.

If the idea of continuous high level alertness appeals to you and you wish to make your own observations you should talk to people who have headache, paroxysmal vertigo or disseminated sclerosis. Outside the neurological field people with coronary thrombosis or peptic ulcer are suitable. Disseminated sclerosis is of particular interest since it affords the opportunity of correlating fluctuations of nervous activity with the onset and fluctuations of the disease. It is worth noting here that it is characteristic of psychosomatic disorders that they are episodic and fluctuating, provided of course the pathology by its nature is reversible. All doctors advise patients with disseminated sclerosis to take a certain amount of rest and you should therefore ask such patients how they put this advice into operation. You will be intrigued to find that to patients rest means muscular rest. However, you should not be too hard on such patients and think them stupid for you will find that the idea of nervous rest is totally foreign to most doctors.

CHAPTER XXXII

THE ELECTRO-ENCEPHALOGRAM

THE electro-encephalogram, or the EEG to use an abbreviation for both the apparatus and the tracing, consists of a series of amplifiers, usually eight, connected to ink-writing units. The amplifiers are connected to electrodes which are attached to the patient's scalp. The EEG is written on paper which moves through the apparatus.

The tracing obtained from the posterior half of the head consists of fairly rhythmic waves, called *alpha* waves, which vary by only half a cycle in individual subjects but between individuals may vary between 8 and 13 cycles per second (CPS). The frequency of the waves is the most important clinical aspect of the EEG although voltage and shapes of waves have also to be taken into account. For convenience in clinical work the range of frequencies is divided into bands as follows.

Less than 4 CPS	4-7 CPS	8-13 CPS	over 13 CPS
delta	*theta*	*alpha*	*beta*

An EEG may consist largely of one frequency, or of different frequencies at different times, or of a mixture of frequencies superimposed on each other.

Types of EEGs

EEGs may be divided into three main types.

1. *Normal EEG.*—This type consists mostly of *alpha* waves and is found in the majority of healthy subjects and in many patients.

2. *Abnormal EEG.*—This type contains delta waves or consists largely of theta waves. It is never found in healthy people. This type may be further divided in terms of the degree of slowing of the waves and in terms of the episodic or continuous nature of such waves but such a division need not concern us here.

   An analysis of abnormal EEGs takes into account the slowness of the waves and their voltage for the slower the waves and the higher the voltage the more abnormal the record. The analysis also takes into account the distribution of the slow activity and three main distributions may be enumerated.

   (*a*) Diffuse and symmetrical between the two hemispheres.

   (*b*) Diffuse and asymmetrical. The term 'asymmetrical' means that the slow waves are more marked in one hemisphere or are confined to one hemisphere.

   (*c*) Focal, that is, the slow waves are most marked in a part of one hemisphere or are confined to that part.

3. *Doubtfully abnormal EEG.*—There is a certain amount of variation in the EEGs of normal sub-

jects and about 10-15 per cent. occupy a position intermediate between the two types already described. An inference of an organic lesion from one EEG of this intermediate type has therefore a very low probability. However, when EEGs are repeated over a period of time and the tracings change from the normal type to the intermediate type, the probability of an organic lesion rises.

EEGs as inferences

Reference has already been made to the two kinds of knowledge in clinical medicine. Here are EEG examples.

People with a cerebral glioma $\xrightarrow{\dfrac{95}{100}}$ have an abnormal EEG.

People with an abnormal EEG $\xrightarrow{\dfrac{1}{1000}}$ have a cerebral glioma.

In the first proposition the EEG is used as an inference. The literature on EEGs contains a vast number of propositions of this type. Such propositions are of doubtful value to the clinician and rather than repeat them some generalisations will be attempted as follows.

1. The more rapidly evolving a histological lesion the more likely is the EEG to be abnormal.

2. The more diffuse the lesion the more likely is the EEG to be abnormal.

3. The more severe the signs the more likely is the EEG to be abnormal.

4. The more rapidly evolving a histological lesion the more likely are abnormal EEGs to precede clinical signs.

These generalisations, although dogmatically stated, lack precision for the term ' *more likely* ' is not very informative with regard to probabilities. The corollaries you may formulate yourself.

In predicting EEGs the best method is to combine the type of lesion and the severity of the signs. For example, it could be safely said that a patient with a glioma *and* a substantial hemiplegia will almost certainly have an abnormal EEG. And in this statement the term ' glioma ' may be replaced by meningitis, encephalitis, abscess and cerbrovascular accident in their early stages; and the term ' hemiplegia ' may be replaced by one or other of the neuro-psychological signs.

It is a good practice to predict EEGs, and indeed the result of any special investigation, for if your predictions are frequently wrong you will be forced to realise that you are not well informed. On the other hand, each of your infrequent errors constitutes valuable evidence. At the risk of confusing you it may be added that a correctly predicted EEG will produce little change in the probabilities of organic inferences. The reason you should try to work out for yourself.

EEGs as evidence

It is obvious that, in clinical practice, EEGs constitute evidence and that to use an EEG clinically is to make inferences from it.

203

Inferences from X-ray appearances alone often have a high probability and, if the X-rays are repeated at intervals, the probability may be very high. Possibly because X-rays and EEGs both use electricity many people suppose that the inferences from EEGs should be within the same high range of probability as that obtained with X-rays. Nothing could be further from the truth. The EEGs obtained from a wide variety of pathologies are roughly similar and it follows that inferences of type of pathology have a low probability. Consequently EEGs should only be used by *adding* them to other clinical evidence with the aim of raising or lowering probabilities. Even with this method the changes in probabilities are, as a rule, not very great. Since EEGs should be used to change probabilities by adding them to other evidence, it is necessary that the clinician should be expert both in clinical neurology and electro-encephalography. Unfortunately, few have achieved this dual expertise and, as a result, the advance of knowledge, with regard to the EEG as evidence, has been extremely slow.

EEGs in organic cerebral lesions generally

People with abnormal EEGs in the absence of seizures	often →	have organic cerebral lesions.
People with grossly abnormal EEGs in the absence of seizures	usually* →	have organic cerebral lesions (histological or chemical).

* In these propositions the term 'usually' and 'rarely' mean nearly always and hardly ever, respectively.

People with psychological signs and an abnormal EEG	usually →	have a diffuse organic cerebral lesion.
People with substantial psychological signs (psychosis) and a normal EEG	rarely →	have an organic cerebral lesion.

EEGs in cerebral infections

People with substantial LT signs or neuro-psychological signs and a normal EEG	rarely →	have a cerebral abscess.

In this proposition meningitis and encephalitis may be substituted for abscess.

EEGs in cerebral neoplasms

People with substantial LT signs or neuro-psychological signs and a normal EEG	rarely →	have a cerebral glioma.
People with slight LT signs or neuro-psychological signs; or Mj/C or MP and a normal EEG	sometimes →	have a cerebral glioma.

These propositions may be valid for other types of cerebral neoplasms. It should be noted that, in the absence of aphasia or substantial LT signs, the EEG abnormalities may be symmetrical even in the presence of a focal neoplasm. On the other hand, the EEG usually becomes asymmetrical when aphasia and substantial LT signs develop.

EEGs in cerebrovascular lesions*

People who have a cerebro-vascular lesion and gross bilateral EEG abnormalities $\xrightarrow{\text{usually}}$ die within a few weeks. The few who survive are usually perman-ently disabled.

People who have a cerebro-vascular incident and have unilateral EEG abnormal-ities $\xrightarrow{\text{usually}}$ survive.

EEGs in seizures (Interseizure EEGs)

People who have Mj/Cs or MPs occurring less than 1/W and beginning over the age of 25 years and who have abnormal EEGs $\xrightarrow[10]{7}$ have organic cerebral lesions.

People with seizures other than Mj/C and MP, no matter their frequency and age of onset, and who have an abnormal EEG $\xrightarrow{\text{often}}$ have organic cerebral lesions.

People who have EEG abnormalities called wave and spike $\xrightarrow{\text{rarely}}$ have organic cerebral lesions.

With regard to seizures the following propositions are worth giving although the EEG is used as an inference.

People who have Mj/Cs occurring at least 1/W $\xrightarrow{\text{usually}}$ have diffuse EEG abnormalities.

People who have MPs occurring at least 1/W $\xrightarrow{\text{usually}}$ have EEG abnormal-ities in one or both temporal lobes.

*A lesion may be substituted for the evidence from which it is inferred if its inference has a very high probability.

206

People who have Mj/Cs or MPs occurring less than 1/W and beginning over the age of 25 years   usually ⟶   have normal EEGs.

People with seizures other than Mj/C and MP, no matter their frequency and age of onset,   usually ⟶   have normal EEGs.

except that people with PM or myoclonus   often ⟶   have wave and spike abnormalities.

EEGs are frequently performed on people with seizures although in many the reason is not evident. A predictably abnormal EEG does not change probabilities, unless in very expert hands, and there is therefore some advantage in being able to make predictions. For people who are over the age of 16 years and who have Mj/C or MP, no matter the age of onset, the following scoring system may be used.

$$1/W = 60$$
$$2(25 - \text{age of onset}) - (20 - \text{duration in years}) + 60 + 1/M = 12$$

(onset over the age of 25 makes this factor zero)   (duration over 20 makes this factor zero) $1/Y = 0$

Duration counts from the end of the last remission and a remission is a period of freedom from seizures of one year. A score over 75 and an abnormal EEG allows only a low probability inference of a cerebral organic lesion. On the other hand, a score under 75 and an abnormal EEG changes the probability to 7/10 and this is increased with markedly abnormal EEGs.

207

The EEG must be recorded a clear week after the last seizure, that is, when the frequency is less than 1/W, since some patients without organic cerebral lesions have abnormal EEGs for a few days after a seizure. It follows from these remarks that in the endeavour to raise the probability of an organic lesion the frequency of the patient's seizures should be reduced to less than 1/W by energetic use of anticonvulsant therapy. To stop therapy before an EEG is not only wrong from a clinical point of view, since status may be induced, but also from an EEG point of view. Most clinicians try very hard by one means or another to provoke abnormalities in the EEGs of people with seizures but their reason for this, unless it is to be considered as an EEG exercise, is never made clear.

EEGs in practice

By studying the above propositions the usefulness and limitations of the EEG will become apparent to you. The following remarks sum up the situation and offer further information.

1. In patients with a psychosis the EEG helps to distinguish organic cerebral lesions from functional cerebral disorders. It is only in a recent psychosis that the EEG is likely to be abnormal for pure psychotic states due to encephalitis and toxic states do not persist for long periods of time. The EEG should therefore be reserved as a diagnostic technique for recent psychotic illnesses. The EEG has no place in the diagnosis of psychoneurotic illnesses.

2. When neuro-psychological signs are equivocal and the probability of a cerebral lesion therefore seems low, an abnormal EEG greatly increases the probability. The EEG is most likely to prove helpful in rapidly evolving lesions (neoplastic or infective) rather than in slow lesions (degenerative).

3. When the clinician has elicited only LT motor signs, an abnormal EEG allows him to infer that the lesion is in the cerebrum.

4. The EEG often indicates the site of a cerebral lesion. The EEG will localise about 75 per cent. of neoplasms but, unfortunately, it is roughly the same 75 per cent. which can be located by bedside examination. This is the reason why neurosurgeons remain unmoved in the face of the apparently impressive claims made by EEG enthusiasts. It is worth mentioning at this point that a focal EEG abnormality slightly raises the probability of a focal lesion as opposed to a diffuse one but it rarely changes the probability of one kind of focal lesion as opposed to another.

5. The EEG has excellent prognostic value for death and survival in cerebrovascular lesions. The number of cases, however, in which it is of more value than bedside examination is small.

6. A single EEG is rarely of value in distinguishing one kind of histological lesion from another. Occasionally, when the EEG abnormalities are in excess of the clinical signs, it may be concluded that a rapid lesion is more likely than a slow one. This balancing of EEGs against signs, however, requires considerable experience. Serial EEGs are occasionally helpful since

progression or regression may be evident while the clinical signs are remaining stationary. In those circumstances the probabilities of progressive or regressive lesions respectively are, of course, raised.

The EEG is occasionally useful in distingishing a histological lesion from a chemical one for with the latter the slow waves have a rather rhythmic appearance which is absent with histological lesions. A focal EEG abnormality, too, considerably raises the probability of a histological lesion as opposed to a chemical one.

7. The EEG in people with seizures has value only in the following fairly unusual circumstances.

(a) When there is a suspicion of a cerebral organic lesion.

(b) When the description of seizures does not allow a clear distinction to be drawn between PMs and MPs and between Mj/Cs and Mj/N-Cs. It is only rarely that such distinctions cannot be drawn on the basis of history-taking and to use the EEG frequently for this purpose is to abuse the technique.

(c) When the frequency of MPs cannot be established since the patient is not always aware of having them. EEG temporal lobe abnormalities indicate that a patient is either having frequent MPs or that there is a temporal lobe lesion. When age, duration or possibly neuro-radiology makes a lesion unlikely it may be concluded that the patient is having frequent MPs.

The EEG cannot be used to identify types of seizures for the type of seizure cannot be inferred from the type of EEG. Exceptions are noted above and even in these, considerable caution is recommended. Most, if not all, clinicians claim that the EEG is useful in diagnosing epilepsy but this claim is worthless for it is not made clear whether epilepsy is an inference (and if it is, what its appearance is) or whether an abnormal EEG is part of the definition of epilepsy. The EEG, without doubt, can be used intelligently in people with seizures without using the term 'epilepsy'. Lastly, it should be noted that anticonvulsant treatment should rarely be influenced by the EEG for, as indicated above, many patients requiring treatment have normal EEGs while many patients with seizures and with abnormal EEGs require something more than anti-convulsant therapy. Furthermore, in patients with seizures who have predictably abnormal EEGs there is sufficient clinical evidence, apart from the EEG, upon which to base drug therapy.

Conclusion

The above remarks on the EEG are of necessity superficial but they should nevertheless give you some insight into this diagnostic technique. Remember, always have some idea of the probabilities of organic inferences before you ask for an EEG to be performed on one of your patients and never ask for the test when organic inferences are extremely low. There is nothing more calculated to kill the enthusiasm of a clinician specialising in EEGs than to be faced with numerous EEGs which are not only normal but are confidently expected to be normal.

CHAPTER XXXIII

THE INCIDENCE AND DIAGNOSIS OF NEUROLOGICAL DISORDERS

THE incidence of neurological disorders is impossible to determine but the relative incidence, based on attendances at a neurological out-patient clinic, is easily given, albeit in crudely approximate terms. In Figure 69 patients are placed in five groups (A, B, C, D and E) on the basis of clinical evidence.

Group A, by far the largest group, consists of patients with paroxysmal disorders (lasting less than six hours) which are given medical names. Major convulsive and non-convulsive and psychical seizures are much the most common. Facial pain and petit mal are relatively rare, while vertigo occupies an intermediate position. Headache (which is very common), whether paroxysmal, episodic or continuous, is included in this group.

Patients are placed in this group because the nature of their symptoms, the age of onset and the absence of physical signs (between the paroxysmal symptoms) make an organic lesion unlikely. It may be taken as a rule that the later the age of onset the more probable is an organic lesion,* except in the case of tic douloureux, although it is not until the onset is in the

* We are thinking, at the moment, in terms of progressive lesions so that traumatic and congenital lesions are excluded.

fifth decade or later that the probability reaches a working level as far as the specialist is concerned. The large number of patients in this group is, no doubt, a reflection of the fact that the majority of patients referred to a neurological out-patient clinic are young or have had their symptoms for long periods.

It is important to note, with regard to this group, that a diagnostic term is a name for evidence. It follows that diagnostic skill consists of an ability to interrogate patients and witnesses, and a knowledge of definitions. Failure to realise the importance of definitions causes the clinician to make heavy weather of his use of diagnostic terms, although it must be added that an obsession with pseudo words such as abnormal discharge and with terms which signify both an effect and its cause contributes its quota to the clinician's confusion.

Group B consists of patients with paroxysmal symptoms of a type which cannot be included in Group A. These do not have medical names and include such symptoms as faintness, lightheadedness, queer feelings and so on.

Group C consists of patients with episodic or continuous symptoms (lasting more than six hours) which allow only a very low probability inference of an organic lesion. Such symptoms defy description.

Group D consists of patients who present evidence from which a particular type of organic lesion can be inferred with a high probability. These lesions have medical names and it follows that diagnostic terms, in the absence of biopsies, are names for inferences. Diagnostic skill, therefore, consists of an ability to collect evidence and a knowledge of correlative propositions. The patients in this group suffer from cervical spondylosis, disseminated sclerosis, mononeuritis, Parkinsonism, brain tumour, spinal compression, syringomyelia, myasthenia gravis and myopathy. It is worth mentioning here that a group of patients with organic lesions are admitted directly to hospital from their homes without first attending an out-patient clinic and, as would be suspected, they suffer from acute conditions such as cerebrovascular accidents, intracranial tumours, meningitis, polyneuritis, poliomyelitis and encephalitis. The diseases enumerated above are in a rough order of frequency.

Group E consists of patients who present evidence which allows a high probability inference of an organic lesion but only a low probability inference of the type of lesion. About a third of the patients who, on attending as out-patients are confidently diagnosed as having organic lesions, remain undiagnosed with regard to the type of lesion. This proportion may be reduced with in-patient investigation but a confident diagnosis is still not possible in about a fifth of the patients. A failure to make a diagnosis of the type of lesion is generally due to sign-time graphs which are incomplete because of poor histories or which, although complete, are not sufficiently distinctive. Sometimes, too, a failure may be due to a paucity of physical signs. As a rule, graphs become more distinctive with the passage of time and as physical signs become more abundant so that, with careful follow-up, most conditions surrender to the clinician's diagnostic skill. At the same time it must be admitted that some conditions resist diagnosis to the bitter end.

It will be seen that, of patients who attend a neurological out-patient clinic, 70 per cent. are considered to have functional disorders and 30 per cent. to have organic lesions. A patient, of course, may occasionally have both a functional disorder and an organic lesion,

THE INCIDENCE OF NEUROLOGICAL DISORDERS

Group A. Paroxysmal symptoms and signs with medical names. Diagnostic terms are names for evidence.	50%	
Group B. Paroxysmal symptoms without medical names	15%	Functional disorders of the nervous system. 70%
Group C. Episodic and continuous symptoms without medical names.	5%	
Group D. Evidence which allows a high probability inference of type of organic lesion.	20%	Organic lesions of the nervous system. 30%
Group E. Evidence which allows a high probability inference of an organic lesion but not of a type of lesion.	10%	

Continuous functional symptoms following trauma are not included.

Fig. 69

for the conditions are not mutually exclusive. The combination, it must be said, calls for the highest diagnostic skill. It should be noted with regard to this combination that Figure 69 is not a classification for, if it were, a patient could not be put into two classes at the one time. The figure is, in fact, no more than a statement of the relative incidence of neurological disorders.

The distinction between a functional disorder and an organic lesion is probably the most important point in clinical medicine and is the source of most confusion and errors. It is unfortunate that the student emerges from his medical school ill-prepared to diagnose functional disorders. The reasons are that clinical teaching is almost entirely concerned with in-patients suffering from organic lesions; that certain functional disorders (Groups B and C) do not lend themselves to clear descriptions; and that certain disorders (Group A) have names which teachers take little trouble to define precisely in terms signifying appearances.

APPENDIX

The CSF in intracranial diseases

In a medical unit the CSF should only be examined in patients suspected of having an infective condition or subarachnoid haemorrhage. A rise of protein without a corresponding rise of cells may be found with an intracranial neoplasm but with this type of lesion a lumbar puncture is dangerous since coning may be produced. Furthermore, a normal protein level, like a normal pressure reading, scarcely reduces the probability of a neoplasm. When, on routine neurological examination, an intracranial neoplasm seems to have a fairly high probability the right course is to proceed directly to neuro-radiology.

You will learn a good deal about CSF changes in your course on infectious diseases. Briefly, several thousand polymorphonuclear cells/cm. may be found in meningococcal, pneumococcal and staphylococcal meningitis, while two or three hundred lymphocytes/cm. may be found in tubercular and viral meningitis and in viral and spirochaetal encephalitis (GPI).

The CSF sugar and chloride levels fall with most infections except those due to a virus. A fall in the sugar level is therefore a useful finding in tubercular meningitis since the CSF cellular changes are similar to those of viral infections. The CSF protein is frequently raised with infections but as a rule this adds little additional information to that already obtained from the changes in cells and sugar.

Bacteriological methods have, of course, to be brought into play when an intracranial infection is being investigated

217

and the WR should be tested whenever neuro-syphilis is a possibility.

The ESR

The ESR is a useful test in neurology since it is rarely raised to any degree in primary diseases of the nervous system (apart from infections) while it is frequently raised to a marked degree in diseases such as carcinoma and periarteritis nodosa which may affect the nervous system secondarily. In other words, a high ESR indicates the need to search outside the nervous system for the primary cause of the neurological lesion. However, it should be noted that cystitis and bed-sores, both of which are common complications of nervous diseases, may cause a substantial rise in the ESR and such a rise has, of course, no diagnostic significance. With regard to bed-sores the ESR rises when the tissues become necrotic, that is, before an ulcer is formed, and the cause of the high ESR may be overlooked unless a careful search is made. When the necrotic tissue sloughs the ESR falls and even with a very large bed-sore the ESR may be only slightly raised. Ignorance of these points may lead you to mis-diagnose a benign condition such as a prolapsed disk.

Radiology of the head

Straight X-rays of the skull are seldom informative although their use cannot be avoided when space-occupying lesions are suspected. The pineal gland is calcified in some people so that a shift of the mid-line structures in an antero-posterior view may be evident. Erosion of the clinoids of the pituitary fossa is sometimes found when increased intra-cranial pressure is fairly long standing although in this event papilloedema, which is nearly always present, has already

218

indicated the increase of pressure. Enlargement of the pituitary fossa, of course, indicates the presence of a pituitary tumour. Some neoplasms, such as a craniopharyngioma, show a degree of calcification and consequently they may be revealed by straight X-rays.

There are several special neuro-radiological techniques, the most important of which is angiography. In this technique a radio-opaque substance is rapidly injected into the carotid or vertebral artery and a series of films taken so that the arterial, capillary and venous circulation are revealed. Displacement of the larger blood vessels is good evidence of a space-occupying lesion, the site of which can readily be inferred. Occasionally, too, the vascular pattern of a neoplasm allows its pathology to be identified. Angiography is of great value in the diagnosis of vascular disorders, for partial and complete stenosis of arteries, aneurysms and vascular tumours may all be demonstrated.

Angiography is occasionally negative with gliomata which, by infiltrating round the vessels may produce little displacement, and frequently negative with deep lesions in the neighbourhood of the ventricles. In these circumstances a ventriculography is performed. In this technique the CSF in the ventricles is partly replaced by air which passes into the lateral ventricles through a cannula inserted in a burr-hole. By exposing films with the head in various positions all parts of the ventricular system can be seen. Thus displacement, enlargement, distortion and blockage of the ventricular system may be demonstrated and from these appearances the site of space-occupying lesions may be inferred with a very high probability. There are some dangers attached to ventriculography, especially when there is increased intracranial pressure, and the technique is therefore strictly reserved for neurosurgeons.

Occasionally a technique called air-encephalography is used. In this, CSF is replaced by air which may be injected into the lumbar subarachnoid space or into the cisterna magna. By this means air not only passes into the ventricles but into the subarachnoid space over the cerebrum so that atrophy of the cerebrum can be diagnosed. The technique should certainly not be used when there is a possibility of a space-occupying lesion since coning may result. The technique, in fact, should be reserved for the diagnosis of degenerative conditions except in special circumstances in a neurosurgical unit.

The reliability of probabilities*

You will remember that cause was defined as a property which, when added or removed, raised or lowered respectively the probability of another property called the effect. Establishing a property as a cause, therefore, entails comparing two probabilities (or proportions) and determining by statistical calculation that a difference between them is unlikely to be fortuitous. A comparison of two probabilities, however, is only valid provided each probability is reliable.

The meaning of the term 'reliability' with regard to probability is made clear by reference to an example. Let us suppose that we have observed 100 men with red hair and have found that 70 per cent. were bad-tempered. May we predict that, of every group of red-haired men observed in the future, 70 per cent. will be bad-tempered? Commonsense rejects this prediction for it seems almost certain that between one group of red-haired men and another there will be substantial differences in the probability of bad

* The probabilities at present considered are of the empirical type. The term 'reliability' could not be appropriately applied to logical probabilities, that is, to probabilities calculated on the basis of certain assumptions.

220

temper. In our present example, therefore, the probability would seem to be unreliable.

It is evident, when we consider the problem, that we have some means of estimating reliability, for we readily judge some probabilities to be reliable and others not. Should we analyse our methods we find that there are three factors in a correlative proposition which influence reliability and these are:

1. The strength of the analogy between the objects of a proposition.
2. The precision of the definition of terms signifying properties.
3. The number of objects observed.

This can be shown in a diagrammatic way.

$$\text{Objects called } A \text{ which have } x \xrightarrow[m]{n} \text{ have } y$$

precision of definitions

strength of analogy   number of objects

The terms 'high' and 'low reliability' are, of course, relative terms, and to avoid misunderstanding it is advisable to make the following statements.

The stronger the analogy; the more precise the definitions; the greater the numbers,	the more reliable the probability.
The weaker the analogy; the less precise the definitions; the smaller the numbers,	the less reliable the probability.

Here are two propositions which have unreliable probabilities.

| vague definitions |

$$\text{Animals which are anxious} \xrightarrow{\frac{5}{8}} \text{are restless}$$

weak analogy   small number

People who have a mild Bell's palsy and who take aspirin several times a day $\xrightarrow{\frac{90}{100}}$ soon show some improvement.

fairly strong analogy

Here, on the other hand, is a proposition which has a highly reliable probability.

People who have pneumonia and are treated with a million units of crystalline penicillin twice daily for a week $\xrightarrow{\frac{90}{100}}$ are afebrile at the end of a week.

Sometimes a probability judged to be reliable turns out to be very unreliable. For example, the probability of 90 per cent. in the last proposition may change to 70 per cent. in a second investigation. If this happened we would, of course, try to account for the discrepancy and we may perhaps find that the ages of the patients in the two investigations were different or that the treatment was started in a different phase of the illness in the two investigations. A probability may therefore prove to be unreliable because relevant evidence is missing from x.

To increase the reliability of the probabilities contained in his propositions the clinician should pay attention to the following points.

1. He should make his definitions as precise as possible and he should use as large numbers as possible. The reason for this you should work out for yourself.

2. He should include in x all the properties which he *knows* alters the probabilities.

3. He should alter the strength of the analogy between his patients.

(*a*) He may strengthen the analogy by choosing only patients who have certain properties, the properties being of a kind which he *speculates* may alter probabilities. Thus, if a clinician speculates that sex alters the probability contained in a proposition, he would arrange that the patients specified in his proposition were all of the same sex. There are many properties in clinical medicine which often alter probabilities and these should be kept in mind in designing an investigation. Such properties are age, sex, weight, social and occupational environments and so on. Rather than select patients with certain properties, the clinician may, of course, strengthen the analogy by selecting patients who do not have certain properties.

It is obvious that, by selecting patients in order to strengthen the analogy, it is possible, provided the method of selection is clearly specified, to repeat the investigation on patients who are very similar to those of the first investigation. As a result the alteration of probabilities by properties not specified under x occurs (or is likely to occur) to the same degree in each investigation and the probabilities are therefore substantially the same in each investigation.

(*b*) Since the selection of patients implies a reduction of the number observed, the clinician is in something of a predicament. However, if he concludes that large numbers are more important than the strength of the analogy, he may intentionally weaken the analogy by selecting patients at random. It should be noted that no choice of patients is completely random and that in the present context we are referring only to the random selection of certain properties such as age, sex, weight and so on. This random selection increases the reliability of a probability because, when the investigation is repeated with patients again selected at random, the incidence of certain properties and the incidence of certain combinations of properties will (or are likely to) match the first investigation fairly well.* Thus, the alteration of probabilities by properties not specified under x occurs (or is likely to occur) to the same degree in each investigation and the probability consequently remains substantially unchanged. It should be noted that methods (a) and (b) are not mutually exclusive, for the analogy may be strengthened with regard to certain properties and weakened with regard to others.

It is obvious that, with regard to the reliability of probabilities, the laboratory worker has a much easier time than the clinician since the former can arrange that there is an extremely strong analogy between his objects of study and he can also arrange that his definitions are extremely precise by introducing accurate quantitative methods. The laboratory worker, too, is fortunate because, with a very strong analogy and very precise definitions, the number observed can be reduced to two or three. The unfortunate clinician, on the other hand, can rarely escape from the necessity of observing large numbers.

By this stage you will perhaps agree that good statistical methods are wasted on unreliable probabilities. You may want to go further and declare that, since the reliability of probabilities can never be reduced to mathematical terms, the validity of statistical methods must sometimes remain a matter of doubt.

* In propositions formulated to establish a cause, the matching of the two series of patients, although partly based on random selection, should be carefully scrutinised.